BIOLOGICAL RHYTHMS AND ENDOCRINE FUNCTION

ADVANCES IN EXPERIMENTAL MEDICINE AND BIOLOGY

Recent Volumes in this Series

BIOLOGICAL RHYTHMS AND ENDOCRINE FUNCTION

Edited by

Laurence W. Hedlund
Department of Dairy Husbandry
University of Missouri
Columbia, Missouri

John M. Franz
Department of Biochemistry
University of Missouri
Columbia, Missouri

and

Alexander D. Kenny
Department of Pharmacology and Toxicology
University of Texas Medical Branch
Galveston, Texas

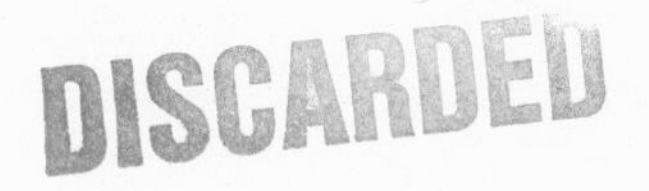

PLENUM PRESS • NEW YORK AND LONDON

Library of Congress Cataloging in Publication Data

Midwest Conference on Endocrinology and Metabolism, 9th,
University of Missouri–Columbia, 1973.
Biological rhythms and endocrine function.

(Advances in experimental medicine and biology; v. 54.)
Includes bibliographical references and index.
1. Biology–Periodicity–Congresses. 2. Glands, Ductless–Congresses. I. Hedlund, Laurence W., ed. II. Franz, John Matthias, 1927- ed. III. Kenny, Alexander D., ed. IV. Dalton Research Center. V. Title. VI. Series. [DNLM: 1. Biological clocks–Congresses. 2. Endocrine glands–Physiology–Congresses. W3 M1307E 1973b/WK102 M629 1973b]
QH527.M52 1973 574.1 74-23448
ISBN 0-306-39054-X

Proceedings of the Ninth Midwest Conference on Endocrinology and Metabolism held at the University of Missouri, Columbia, Missouri, October 18-19, 1973 and sponsored by

University of Missouri– Columbia
  Dalton Research Center
  Extension Division
  Graduate School
  Graduate Student Association
  School of Medicine
  School of Veterinary Medicine
  Sinclair Comparative Medicine Research Farm
Ciba-Geigy Corporation
Merck, Sharp and Dohme
Organon Incorporated
Ortho Research Foundation
G. D. Searle and Company
E. R. Squibb and Sons Incorporated
The Upjohn Company

A Division of Plenum Publishing Corporation
227 West 17th Street, New York, N.Y. 10011

United Kingdom edition published by Plenum Press, London
A Division of Plenum Publishing Company, Ltd.
4a Lower John Street, London, W1R 3PD, England

Printed in the United States of America

Conference Chairman

Alexander D. Kenny, Ph.D., *Professor of Biochemistry and Investigator, Dalton Research Center, University of Missouri — Columbia.*

Planning Committee

William C. Allen, M.D., *Associate Medical Director of Medical Center, Associate Professor of Community Health and Medical Practice, University of Missouri — Columbia.*

Ralph R. Anderson, Ph.D., *Associate Professor of Dairy Husbandry, University of Missouri — Columbia.*

Gail I. Bank, Ph.D., *Executive Director of Continuing Medical Education, Associate Professor of Extension Education, University of Missouri — Columbia.*

Robert P. Breitenbach, Ph.D., *Professor of Biological Sciences, University of Missouri — Columbia.*

Billy N. Day, Ph.D., *Professor of Animal Husbandry, University of Missouri — Columbia.*

Horst-Dieter Dellmann, Dr. med. vet., Ph.D., *Professor of Veterinary Anatomy, University of Missouri — Columbia.*

Mostafa S. Fahim, Ph.D., *Associate Professor of Obstetrics and Gynecology, University of Missouri — Columbia.*

Franklin W. Figg and James O. Preston, *Conference Coordinators, Conferences and Short Courses, University Extension Division, University of Missouri — Columbia.*

John M. Franz, Ph.D., *Associate Professor of Biochemistry, University of Missouri — Columbia.*

Laurence W. Hedlund, Ph.D., *Assistant Professor of Dairy Husbandry, University of Missouri — Columbia.*

J. Alan Johnson, Ph.D., *Assistant Professor of Physiology, University of Missouri — Columbia*

David M. Klachko, M.D., *Assistant Professor of Medicine, University of Missouri— Columbia.*

X. J. Musacchia, Ph.D., *Professor of Physiology and Investigator, Dalton Research Center, University of Missouri — Columbia.*

William P. Palmore, D.V.M., Ph.D., *Associate Professor of Veterinary Physiology, University of Missouri — Columbia.*

Arnold A. White, Ph.D., *Associate Professor of Biochemistry and Investigator, Dalton Research Center, University of Missouri — Columbia.*

Speakers

Roger A. Gorski, Ph.D., *Professor of Anatomy, Center for the Health Sciences, University of California, Los Angeles, California.*

Franz Halberg, M.D., *Professor of Pathology, Chronobiology Laboratories, Health Sciences Center, University of Minnesota, Minneapolis, Minnesota.*

Julian I. Kitay, M.D., *Professor of Internal Medicine and Physiology, University of Virginia School of Medicine, Charlottesville, Virginia.*

Dorothy T. Krieger, M.D., *Professor of Medicine, Mount Sinai School of Medicine of the City University of New York, New York.*

Harry J. Lynch, Ph.D., *Research Associate, Department of Nutrition and Food Science, Massachusetts Institute of Technology, Cambridge, Massachusetts.*

Russel J. Reiter, Ph.D., *Associate Professor of Anatomy, University of Texas Medical School, San Antonio, Texas.*

E. P. Wallen, Ph.D., *Department of Physiology and Cell Biology, University of Kansas, Lawrence, Kansas.*

J. M. Yochim, Ph.D., *Department of Physiology and Cell Biology, University of Kansas, Lawrence, Kansas.*

Moderators

Horst-Dieter Dellmann, Dr. med. vet., Ph.D., *Professor of Veterinary Anatomy, University of Missouri — Columbia.*

James A. Green, Ph.D., *Professor of Anatomy, University of Missouri — Columbia.*

Laurence W. Hedlund, Ph.D., *Assistant Professor of Dairy Husbandry, University of Missouri — Columbia.*

J. Alan Johnson, Ph.D., *Assistant Professor of Physiology, University of Missouri — Columbia.*

Discussants

Craig, B. W., *Wichita State University, Wichita, Kansas.*

Dellmann, H.-D., *Department of Veterinary Anatomy, University of Missouri — Columbia.*

Franz, J. M., *Department of Biochemistry, University of Missouri — Columbia.*

Friend, L. J., *College of Medicine, University of Nebraska, Omaha, Nebraska.*

Hedlund, L. W., *Department of Dairy Husbandry, University of Missouri — Columbia.*

Jackson, G., *College of Veterinary Medicine, University of Illinois, Urbana, Illinois.*

Karsch, F., *Department of Pathology, University of Michigan, Ann Arbor, Michigan.*

Prahlad, K. V., *Department of Biological Sciences, Northern Illinois University, Dekalb, Illinois.*

Ramaley, J., *Department of Physiology and Biophysics, University of Nebraska Medical Center, Omaha, Nebraska.*

Sellner, R., *University of Missouri — Kansas City, Kansas City, Missouri.*

Preface

These Proceedings of the Midwest Conference on Endocrinology and Metabolism are being published by Plenum Press for the first time. Earlier Proceedings in the series were published by the University of Missouri at Columbia. The shift to an internationally recognized publisher reflects the considerable growth in stature that the Midwest Conferences have undergone since their inception nine years ago. Originally concerned only with the endocrinology of the thyroid, the Conferences now explore other endocrine areas. Efforts are made to assemble a panel of speakers selected from different sub-disciplines within endocrinology for the purpose of addressing a common problem. The Ninth Conference typifies this approach.

The format used in recent Conferences is not unique, but is unfortunately encountered too rarely. A few prominent scholars are invited to come together to expound their findings and concepts in considerable depth, and to participate in a discussion which, together with the formal presentation, is published in the Proceedings. The discussion, noted for its unhurried nature, permits wide participation by the audience.

The subject of the Ninth Conference is one which is basic and important not only to endocrinology but also to biology in general. Many, possibly most, life processes change in a rhythmic fashion, with similar states recurring at regular time intervals. This rhythmic property of living systems expresses itself as a recognizable and definable pattern or "time-form" in a manner equivalent to the more customary spatial-form.

Traditionally, biologists have given major attention to problems relating to spatial-form; and we now have reached a point where we can comfortably comprehend the whole animal in terms of how various subcomponents fit together in three dimensional space. We also realize that patterns of process or change that occur within animals at the molecular, micro-, and macro-levels must also fit together in a similarly meaningful fashion to give form in the time dimension. However, critical description and analysis of "time-form" is a more recent development, and we are now beginning to appreciate the magnitude of complexity of living systems when considered in terms of this dimension. The Editors and contributors hope that this volume will assist the reader in achieving a useful overview of the "time-form" dimension in general and in relation to several specific endocrine areas.

The Editors wish to thank especially Wanda Wells and the stenographic staff of the Dalton Research Center for the excellent services rendered in producing camera-ready copy for the Publisher. Thanks are also due the Moderators and the other members of the Planning Committee without whose valuable help the Conference could not have succeeded. To the sponsors of the Conference, whose financial support made it a reality, a deep appreciation is felt by the Editors and the Planning Committee.

Laurence W. Hedlund

John M. Franz

Alexander D. Kenny

Contents

BIOLOGICAL RHYTHMS

PINEAL RHYTHMS

GONADAL RHYTHMS

ADRENAL CORTICAL RHYTHMS

BIOLOGICAL RHYTHMS

Franz Halberg

Chronobiology Laboratories
Department of Laboratory Medicine and Pathology
Health Sciences Center
University of Minnesota
Minneapolis, Minnesota 55455

OUTLINE

I. INTRODUCTION

Relativistic Time in Biology and Physics

"Before the advent of the theory of relativity it had always been tacitly assumed in physics that the statement of time had an absolute significance, i.e., that it is independent of the state of motion of the body of reference" (Einstein, 1920, 1922). Einstein challenged the concept of simultaneity for events taking place at a great distance, said to occur at the same moment in some "absolute time." He conceived of time as a coordinate always associated with the three space coordinates for any reference body under consideration in a four-dimensional mani-

Supported by the USPHS (5-K6-GM-13 891), NASA, NCI, Office of Naval Research (1R01-CA-14445-01), and NSF.

fold. To many physicists today time is not absolute, but only a measurement that depends on the frame of reference from which it is made (Einstein, 1920, 1922, 1905). Einstein emphasized that a statement of the time of an event has no meaning unless it is accompanied by an indication of the reference body. (As a consequence he claimed the passage of time is retarded in a system moving at high speed. According to his theory of relativity, events in a high-speed system appear to occur more slowly -- including life processes, notably aging. The problem of whether the passage of time depends upon speed continues to be a subject of experimentation [Hafele and Keating, 1972] as well as debate [Terrell, 1972]).

Just as physicists are concerned with relativistic time biomedical investigators also focus upon the time frame of phenomena studied by them, i.e., upon relative biologic time (Halberg and Simpson, 1967; Halberg, Nelson, Runge, Schmitt, Pitts, Tremor, and Reynolds, 1971).

Man indeed lives and acts in time. He should become aware that there are "schedules" originating within his body (Halberg, 1969) quite apart from those dictated by the environment. We emphasize, in this connection, the feasibility of isolating and quantifying rhythmic aspects of biological time superimposed upon growth, development, and aging (Halberg, 1961; Hellbrügge, 1960; Descovich, Montalbetti, Kühl, Rimondi, and Halberg, 1973; Rummel, Lee, and Halberg, 1974).

Before the advent of objective rhythm assessment, biomedical indications of duration usually were given in conventional time units, timing being given by no more than clock hour and date (if it was not altogether ignored). Such practice presumes an absolute and identical flow of both biologic and clock-calendar time. The fallacy of this line of thought emerges from several kinds of evidence.

Menstrual cycle lengths vary in conventional time units -- by many days -- yet the cycles themselves may be biologically equivalent. Two approximately 24-hour circadian rhythms (from Latin "circa" meaning about, and "dies" meaning 24 hours) may differ consistently from 24 hours in the free-running state; their time relations to each other may remain similar or they may differ from those on a 24-hour-synchronized schedule (Figure 1). A drastic difference in the timing of circadian hormonal changes, expressed in relation to local clock time for natives of an equatorial rain forest and medical students in Glasgow, disappears when these data are referred to the schedule of sleeping and waking of the subjects (Figure 2). The latter time coordinates are internal to the given system under study (Halberg and Simpson, 1967), and their use critically determines the analytical results. We need to focus on the description and quantification of both external and internal physiologic "timing" and thereby attempt, among other tasks, to render learning and teaching processes more motivating and relevant to problems of modern man, his health, and his environment (Halberg, 1973; Halberg, Halberg, Halberg, and Halberg, 1973).

II. BIOLOGIC RHYTHMS

Rhythms are statistical events; in <u>like</u> fashion they recur at <u>similar</u> intervals in <u>comparable</u> sequences. <u>To be</u> rhythmic, the events, <u>the</u>

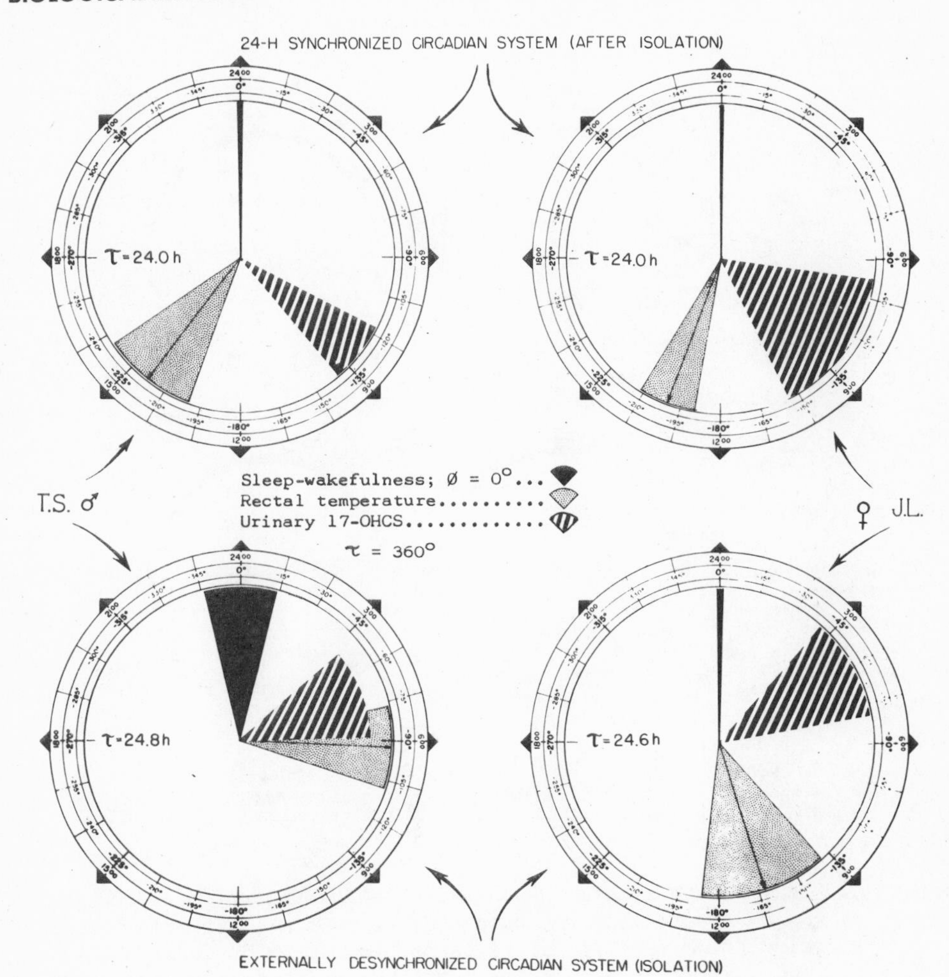

Figure 1. Internal timing with respect to sleep-wakefulness of two human prominent circadian rhythms in the 24-hour synchronized and in an externally desynchronized state. From: Halberg and Reinberg, 1967.

intervals, and the sequences are not necessarily identical but they must show some regularity. To qualify as a rhythm to a chronobiologist the regularity must have an identifiable pattern and must be shown very unlikely to have occurred by chance (Halberg, Nelson, Runge, Schmitt, Pitts, Tremor, and Reynolds, 1971). This condition applies to the heart; it beats at similar yet never consistently identical intervals with a rate that will change as one runs or rests. By the same token, we inhale and exhale in another modifiable rhythm. Equally obvious are the recurring changes from sleep to wakefulness, or menstruation in the healthy mature

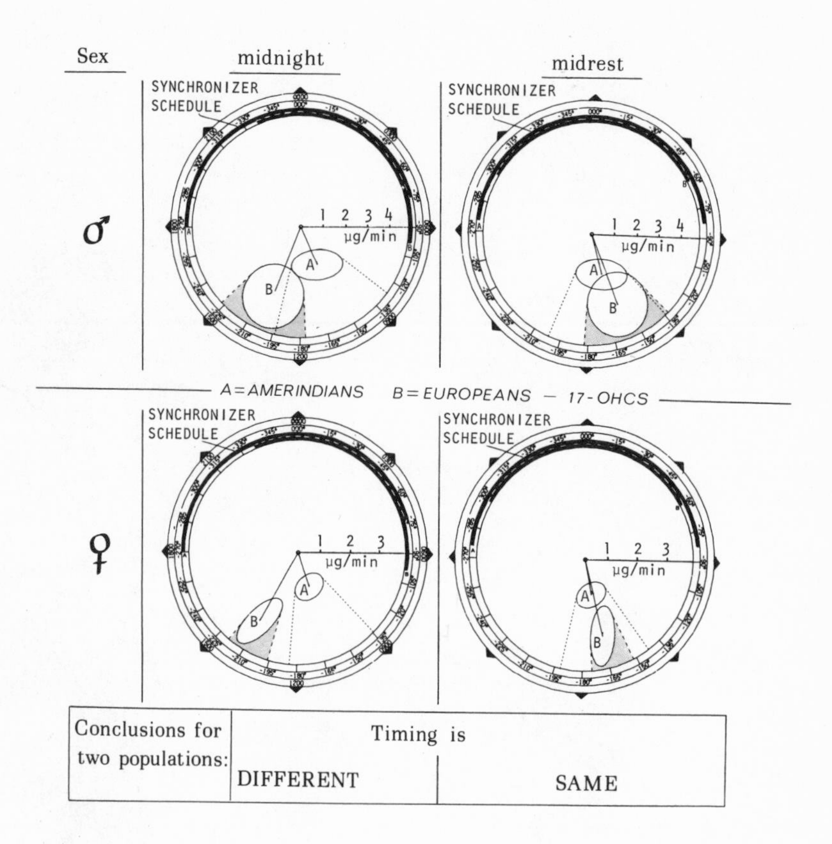

Figure 2. Timing of circadian rhythms in 17-hydroxycorticoid excretion by Europeans and Amerindians differs when it is referred to clock time (left); yet it is the same when it is referred to mid-rest (right). In the cosinor display in the left column, the computative acrophase, ϕ, is the angle formed by a directed line with the acrophase reference at midnight, shown as zero degrees. The amplitude, A, is shown by the length of a directed line. Values for ϕ and A are given in the cosinor displays. The figure reveals a statistically significant rhythm for both the Amerindians and the Europeans. When midnight is used as reference time point, the difference in acrophase is statistically significant for women in view of the nonoverlapping 95 percent confidence arcs. When the reference time point is changed to the middle of the habitual sleep span (right), the internal acrophases no longer differ. Thus, a simple, common-sense adjustment in acrophase reference eliminates a spurious intergroup difference and provides an objective, quantitative, cross-culturally valid index for the timing of an important rhythm in different populations. From: Halberg and Simpson, 1957.

woman. But there are many other biologic rhythms of which we are just becoming aware, if at all.

With appropriate numerical methods and displays, the rhythmic (and thus predictable) part of much biologic variability can be analyzed and isolated. Computer technology thus becomes an important tool for those dealing with the time dimension of biology -- the chronobiologists (Scheving, Halberg, and Pauly, 1974).

Many old observations gain new meaning from modern electronically executed analyses. Several hundred years ago a monthly period in body weight was reported for men (Santorio, 1957). More recently, periods of one or several weeks as well as one month were found in male hormone excretion and performance. These bioperiodicities have been verified and quantified by computer techniques applied to body weight, performance, and hormonal data (Halberg, Engeli, Hamburger, and Hillman, 1965) and await application in biology and medicine, e.g., in accounting for intermittencies of performance and behavior in health as well as for heretofore unexplained time patterns of disease (Reimann, 1963; Halberg, 1968; Simpson, Gjessing, Fleck, Kühl, and Halberg, 1974).

The heartbeat rate is different when we inhale than when we exhale, quite apart from changes related to physical and mental activities. Moreover, the isolated heart deprived of controls continues to beat. The cardiac rhythm is intrinsic to the heart; rhythm is intrinsic to the adrenal gland whether one sleeps or not (Halberg, 1953; Halberg, 1965; Halberg, Frank, Harner, Matthews, Aaker, Gravem, and Melby, 1961; Haus and Halberg, 1962; Ungar and Halberg, 1962; Andrews, 1968; Shiotsuka, Jovonovich, and Jovonovich, 1974). The DNA in the cells (the material that carries genetic information from generation to generation), the rates of cell division, and many features of our biochemical and biophysical makeup also demonstrate circadian rhythmicity (Halberg, Halberg, Barnum, and Bittner, 1959).

III. PERSISTENCE

Studies on the mouse have revealed that the timing of circadian rhythms can be displaced along the 24-hour scale by changes in the lighting and feeding regimens. After blinding, however, these same rhythms persist in many variables, with periods differing slightly from precisely 24 hours and differing also from individual to individual (Aschoff, 1960; Halberg, 1960). In continuous darkness as well, mice maintain several aspects of their circadian time structure. The alternation of light and darkness thus cannot be the sole reason for rhythmicity. For animals in continuous darkness (Halberg, 1960), as well as for those kept in alternating light and darkness (Haus and Halberg, 1959), the same dose of a poison such as ethanol is much more toxic at one time than at another. Many rhythms continue to occur in environmental temperatures kept as constant as is possible with current technology. In these cases changes in temperature -- by night or during winter -- also can be ruled out as accounting for circadian or circannual (approximately yearly) rhythms. The persistence of rhythms in man, too, has been demonstrated in individuals isolated in caves who followed self-selected schedules

(Halberg and Reinberg, 1967; Mills, 1967; Halberg, Reinberg, Haus, Ghata, and Siffre, 1970).

IV. CIRCADIAN RHYTHMS

In usage by participants at a symposium (Pittendrigh, 1960; Aschoff, 1960; Halberg, 1960) the term "circadian" applies to physiologic (average) periods of exactly 24-hour length and to periods that on the average are slightly, yet consistently, shorter or longer than 24 hours by minutes or by a few hours. For instance, circadian may be used to describe the period of either of the two curves shown in Figure 3a. The

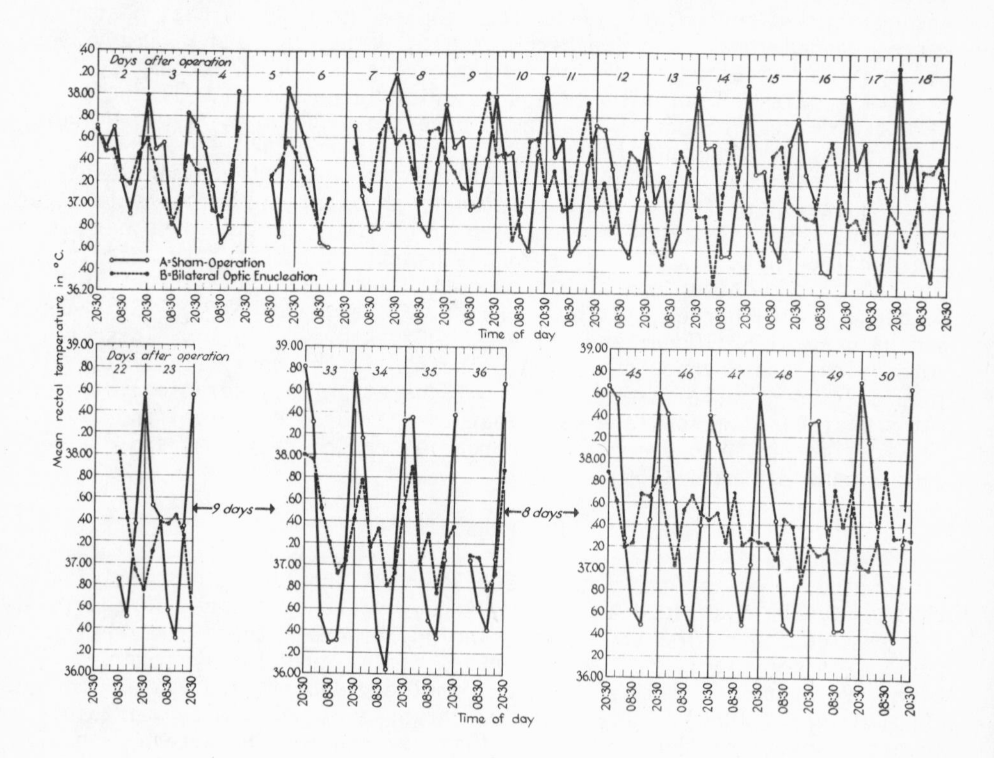

Figure 3a. Bilateral optic enucleation uncoupled the rectal temperature rhythm of male hybrid mice from a cycle of 12 hours of light alternating with 12 hours of darkness. Data plotted as a function of time.

solid line is of average 24-hour length; the dotted line has a mean period of about 23 hours and 20 minutes (see Figure 3b) (Halberg, 1954, 1970).

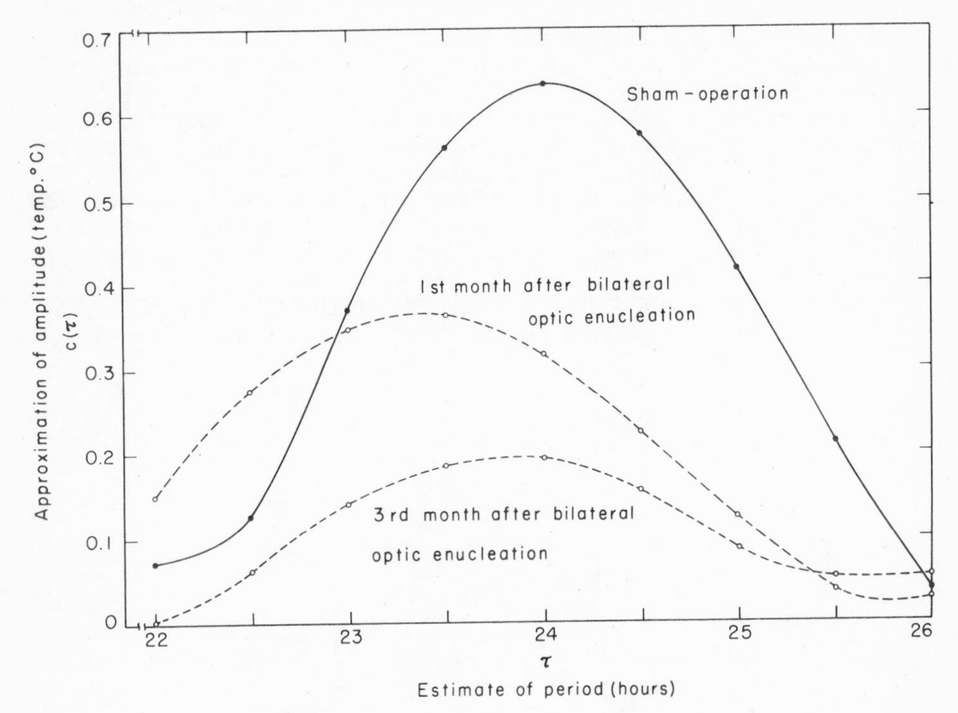

Figure 3b. The analysis of certain data sections from Figure 3a by periodograms are shown here. In a periodogram the point of maximum ordinate provides an estimate of period on the abscissa, provided there is a well-defined maximum point. The periodogram on the data obtained during the first post-operative month from blinded mice reveals a slight shortening of circadian cycle length. A corresponding phase difference between the rhythms in blinded and sham-operated animals can be verified by the large phase difference apparent between the curves plotted simply as a function of time on days 22 and 23 post-operation (see Figure 3a). From: Halberg and Visscher, 1954.

The difference in period is apparent in Figure 3a from the lead in "peak-time" of temperature rhythm in blinded mice; by day 22 this rhythm is roughly in temporary antiphase, in relation to that of sham-operated controls. The average circadian period in rectal temperature of the group of blinded mice is slightly but consistently shorter than 24 hours. We are here dealing with a desynchronization of the circadian rhythm from the 24-hour clock-regulated cycle of 12 hours of light alternating with 12 hours of darkness.

It is methodologically, as well as theoretically, important to recognize circadian periods that differ from exactly 24 hours since, for example, the peak of a given rhythmic function with such a period will occur at a different time each day. Thus, if the period is shorter than 24 hours, the peak will occur earlier each day (dotted lines in Figure 3a) while it will occur later each day if the circadian period is longer than 24 hours.

The abstract Figure 4 serves to emphasize the relevance of circadian system analysis to general biomedical methods whenever circadian

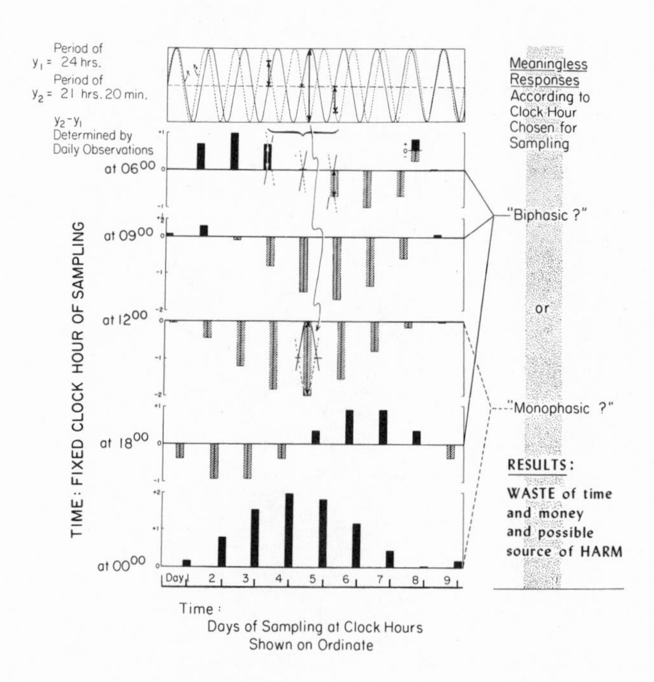

Figure 4. Circadian system physiology is not merely a study of clock-hour effects. Work at a fixed time of day does not forestall disastrous pitfalls possibly invalidating much research on rhythmic functions. This is seen from a study of the time-course of an inter-group difference between synchronized controls and desynchronized experimentals -- when comparisons are made 24 hours apart, at one or the other clock-hour.

In this figure a given physiologic function, y, is assumed to be circadian periodic in both groups compared. y_1 could re-

present a 24-hour-synchronized case, while y_2 could differ in period from y_1 by 160 minutes in time. On the plot, y_1 and y_2 start out in phase at 06^{00} in each case. Note that the difference between the two groups being compared will change drastically with time, as a function of the particular clock-hour chosen for observation.

This figure is intended for authors (and referees!) who, believing that chronobiology is too complex, have "done something about rhythms" by repeating their observations at a conveniently fixed clock-hour. These students may be helped by the recognition that the time-course and sign (!) of an intergroup difference can be rather critically dependent upon the particular clock-hour chosen for study.

In a scientific community at large the timing of observations will, of course, vary with the circadian systems of the investigators and their social schedules. Thus, the abstract Figure 4 may not be unrealistic if it compares the results obtained by several investigators, each working at a fixed time of day with the clock-hour for daily observations differing, however, from one student to the next.

At the identical time, on day 0, each of five investigators performs the same operation or treatment on a group of experimentals, and thereafter observes some physiologic function y_2. Concomitantly, a sham-operation or treatment is done for the study of the same physiologic function, y_1, on a control group. The operations may result in free-running of y_2 but not of y_1. This is shown at the top of Figure 4.

An early-rising student will compare y_1 and y_2 daily at 06^{00} (second row in Figure 4). His post-operative "finding" is an initial rise of the physiologic function above the control level and a subsequent fall below that level. An equally skilled person working at 09^{00} confirms his observation but with some differences in the time-course and extent of change (third row in Figure 4). Both presume that "effects of rhythms" are eliminated since each made his observations on both controls and experimentals at the same clock-hour the same day of the week, or the same time of the year. They are skeptical, of course, when a third equally "competent" investigator of the same functions, y_1 and y_2, working at noon, describes as the result of the same operation an initial fall (not rise!) of the physiologic function in experimentals and a subsequent return to control values.

By now a "monophasic" and two "biphasic" responses are available to describe the same post-operative phenomenon. Yet another "biphasic response" will be recorded by a student working at 18^{00} and it will be rather opposite to that reported by his fellow 06^{00} worker. The "monophasic response" of the man on a midnight shift (bottom of Figure 4), in its turn, will be nearly the reverse of that found during the customary lunch hour.

Results such as those considered in this figure are often complicated by yet other factors. Such "noise" renders most biologic data more complex. Whether or not our research interest includes circadian and other rhythms as such, understanding of circadian or circannual systems seems essential to interpreting one or the other "monophasic" or "biphasic" response to the identical treatment.

The cases here discussed are germane to pharmacology and therapeutics, insofar as animal experiments and clinical trials are concerned. In such endeavors we may record even from healthy subjects responses such as those presented in this figure, notably if we attempt to "control" conditions by instituting, say, constancy in a number of environmental factors such as the lighting regimen for an experimental animal group. In the event that we synchronize our animals, like a human being is synchronized by his social routine, we must also ascertain that the period or phase of a rhythm is the same in both the presence and absence of drug administration or disease. If this is not the case, "responses" such as those in the figure may mislead us to wishing to replace what is superficially believed to be missing (yet is not missing) or to remove what superficially (and wrongly) appears to be excessive. Let us consider more specifically against the background of the figure what may be gained for therapeutic action when the responses shown are used as a basis for judgment and an unevaluated rhythm confounds the results.

The student working daily at noon, who recorded a "drop," e.g., in a biochemical value of his patient, will advocate replacement therapy. This would be disputed (and should be) by his colleague working at midnight, who recorded a "rise" and recommends the opposite treatment.

Were it not that the more prominent and thus more influential investigators of circadian systems are themselves synchronized by rather similar social schedules, disputes would be much more frequent. However, whether or not a "response" is contested matters little; actually, the undisputed "result" is the more dangerous one since it forms the basis of unwarranted clinical action.

We have noted earlier that y_1 *and* y_2*, as computed and drawn for this figure, differ in their circadian period by 160 minutes. The monophasic and biphasic responses thus "occurred" within a few days. Obviously, if the difference in the periods of* y_1 *and* y_2 *is smaller, these responses will be the same in principle but will "occur" more slowly -- after weeks, months, or years. It may be worthwhile, in the future, to see whether any of our "controlled responses" in biology and medicine -- long-term and short-term "phenomena" alike -- are amenable to more meaningful resolution after scrutiny by circadian analysis. Whether or not this be so, the trivial response spectrum of this figure approximates factual observations, as may indirectly become* *apparent from many studies cited or reported at the 1960 Cold Spring Harbor Symposium on Quantitative Biology. From: Halberg, Loewenson, Winter, Bearman, and Adkins, 1960.*

periodic functions susceptible to desynchronization are involved. Figure 4 does so in revealing the pitfalls of interpretation that are unavoidable when circadian system analysis is omitted. A given physiological function (y) is assumed to be circadian periodic in both groups compared. y_1 could represent a 24-hour synchronized case while y_2 could differ in period from y_1 by 160 minutes in time (case 3, desyncrhonization discussed in Halberg, Loewenson, Winter, Bearman, and Adkins, 1960). On the plot, y_1 and y_2 start out with the same values at 06^{00}. Note that the difference between the two groups being compared undergoes drastically different changes with time as a function of the particular clock-hour chosen for observation. Similar patterns are found in a plethora of publications on functions previously demonstrated as circadian periodic, but their value as such seems questionable.

An important reason for the recording of responses in health and disease is our motivation to replace what is missing and to remove what is excessive. Let us consider what we gain for therapeutic action when our judgment rests on responses such as those in Figure 4.

Working daily at noon, one records a "drop," e.g., in a hormonal or other biochemical value of a patient and replacement therapy seems justified. This can be disputed (and should be) by another investigator working at midnight who finds a "rise" and recommends the opposite treatment. Whether or not a "response" is contested matters not; actually, the undisputed "result" is a more dangerous one since it forms the basis of unwarranted and potentially harmful clinical action. In Figure 4, y_1 and y_2 were computed and drawn so as to differ in their circadian period by 160 minutes. The monophasic and biphasic responses thus "occurred" within a few days.

Obviously, if the difference in the periods of y_1 and y_2 is smaller, these responses will be the same in principle but will occur more slowly -- during weeks, months, or years. Responses such as those sketched in Figure 4 are recorded with control as to the time of day but not as to the stage of the circadian system; they are amenable to more meaningful resolution after scrutiny by circadian analysis. Actually, the trivial response spectrum of this figure approximates factual observations (Figure 3a). Figure 3a in turn is hardly a unique curiosity as may become apparent indirectly from important early studies by Aschoff, Pittendrigh, and others reporting at the 1960 Cold Spring Harbor Symposium on Quantitative Biology (Aschoff, 1960; Pittendrigh, 1960; Halberg, 1960).

V. DIURNAL

As described but not prescribed by the Glossary Committee of the International Society for Chronobiology (Halberg, Katinas, Chiba, Garcia-

Sainz, Kovats, Kunkel, Montalbetti, Reinberg, Scharf, and Simpson, 1973) diurnal is not a synonym for circadian. This adjective does not convey the notion that physiological (average) periods can consistently differ in length from exactly 24 hours -- quite apart from the ambiguity which results when, as in the case of diurnal, one and the same term is applied to the entire 24-hour period on the one hand and to "daytime," as opposed for instance to "nighttime," on the other hand. This ambiguity might be eliminated as is suggested in Figure 5.

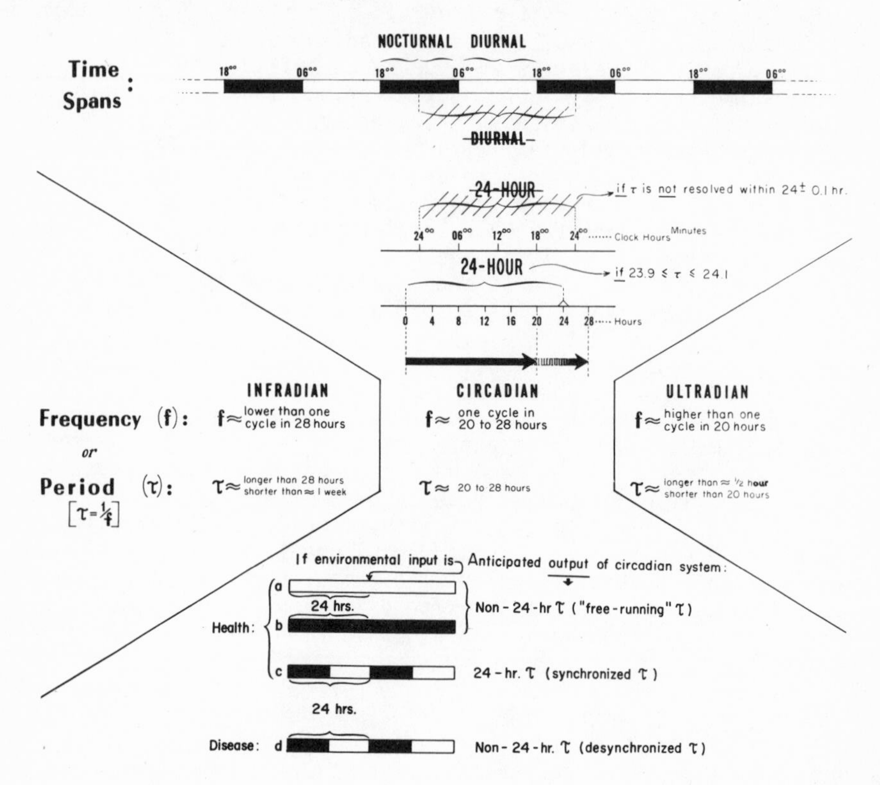

Figure 5. Some terminology used in this paper to describe changes with several frequencies in a given physiologic function. From: Halberg, 1965.

The established uses of diurnal for distinguishing biologic events limited mainly to daytime from those limited to other parts of the 24-hour period, as in diurnal (versus nocturnal) filariasis or epilepsy, or in "diurnality" (versus "nocturnality") of activity patterns suffice, in themselves, as arguments for restricting this adjective to designate the daytime only. This restriction is even more warranted since by refraining from the use of diurnal for designating the entire 24-hour period, one might succeed in removing the image which reference to "diurnal variations" evokes in the minds of many investigators, namely the unqualified association of certain physiological events with certain particular times of day.

VI. ULTRADIAN RHYTHMS

The adjective ultradian can be used to modify a period as well as a frequency. It should be remembered that ultradian is coined with reference to frequency. This coinage is analogous or similar to names applied in physics to certain wavelengths beyond the range of audible sound or visible light, respectively -- the prefix "ultra" denoting a shorter wavelength, i.e., a higher frequency. For instance, "ultrasonic" are mechanical waves of frequencies beyond the range of audibility, and "ultraviolet" are radiations of frequencies next higher than those of the visible violet. The analogy holds for ultrasonic and the similarity for ultraviolet wavelength.

Ultradian near-rhythms usually are wobbling frequencies and are difficult to evaluate by the inspection of original data, such as observations plotted as a function of time. When assessed by variance spectra these near-rhythms stand out as broad bands. The greater their irregularity, the broader the band, i.e., the wider the range of frequencies or periods covered by their estimates on the abscissa (Figures 6 and 7; see qualifications in legends).

If one does not analyze ultradian variation but simply presents undigested data, one may speak of episodic secretion. However, science does, as a rule, require also some ordering. For episodic secretions one can give means and standard errors and ranges as in Table 1. One can also analyze such data as done in Tables 2 and 3, for the case of 17-hydroxycorticosteroid concentration and output, respectively, in canine adrenal venous effluent. If they are statistically prominent components, one can speak of ultradian rhythms rather than ultradian variation and thereby opens an avenue to tour the quantification of ultradian rhythms as these may change from sleep to wakefulness or from the follicular to the luteal stage of the menstrual cycle.

VII. ADRENOCORTICAL PACEMAKER

The adrenal cycle (Halberg and Visscher, 1952; Halberg, 1953; Halberg, Frank, Harner, Matthews, Aaker, Gravem, and Melby, 1961; Halberg, 1965) deserves consideration as an entity that prepares the organism for each day's activities and thus is essential for survival. In a rodent or man certain circadian rhythms depend upon an adrenocortical cycle. Thus, a rhythm in certain blood cell counts, as well as enzymes, mitoses, and urinary electrolytes, is obliterated after adrenal gland removal and reinduced by the periodic administration of adrenal hormones. Dr. Herbert E. Brown of the Department of Anatomy, University of Missouri - Columbia, has done pioneering work while in Utah. He demonstrated dramatically large amplitude rhythms in several blood cell counts,

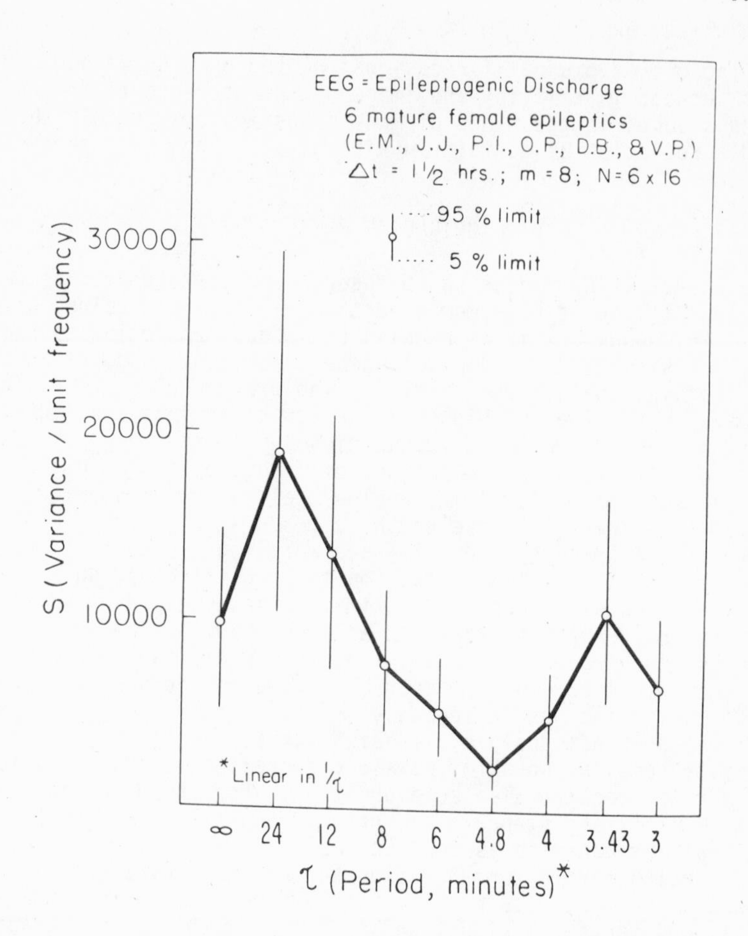

Figure 6. Pooled variance spectrum -- on six series of pathologic electroencephalographic discharge -- may be used for the concomitant exploration of the relative prominence of a circadian component, on the left, and of an ultradian component, with a period of about 3 1/2 hours, on the right. However, both components are too close to the ends of the spectral domain analyzed to allow for a rigorous interpretation. Data recorded at the Cambridge State School and Hospital in Cambridge, Minnesota. The author is indebted to Dr. Rudolf Engel of the University of Oregon at Portland for evaluating the time percent of abnormal discharge or the number of spikes in these records. From: Halberg, 1965.

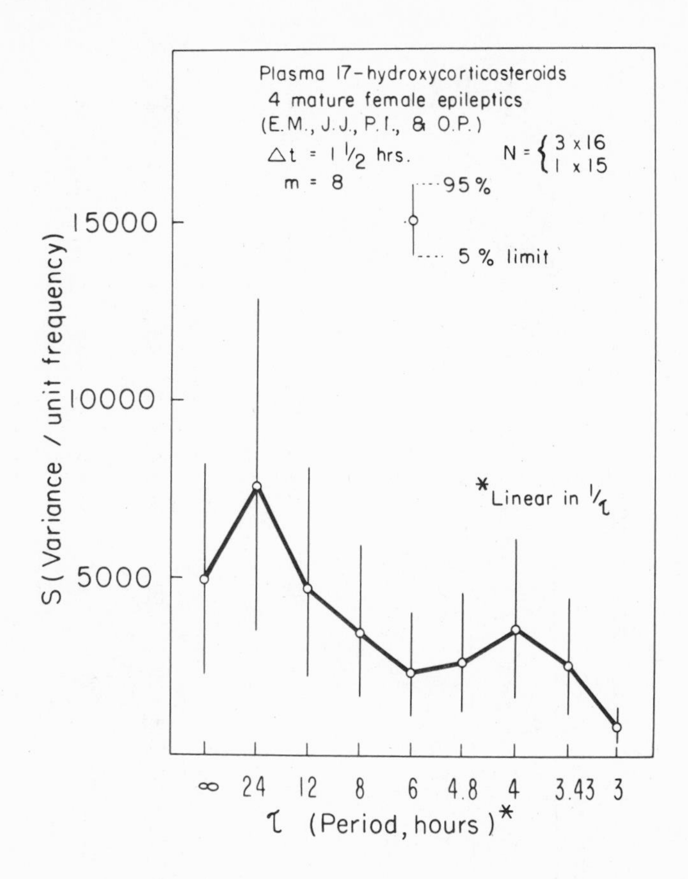

Figure 7. Pooled variance spectrum on four series of plasma 17-hydroxycorticosteroid, for the concomitant exploration of the relative prominence of circadian and ultradian components. The qualifications made in the legend to Figure 6 apply to this analysis as well. The components studied (on these four series, rather than six, as in Figure 6) cannot be ascertained as being statistically significant in view of the "noise level" on hand. Units on ordinate are arbitrary. From: Halberg, 1965.

total counts, lymphocyte counts as well as eosinophil counts, and demonstrated further, as we have found (Halberg, Visscher, Flink, Berge, and Bock, 1951; Halberg, Visscher and Bittner, 1953) that adrenalectomy

Table 1. 17-HYDROXYCORTICOSTEROIDS IN VENOUS ADRENAL EFFLUENT AND ARTERIAL FEMORAL BLOOD OF DOGS INVESTIGATED

Dog No.	Adrenal Effluent						Arterial Blood		
	Output (μg/min)			Concentration (μg %)			Concentration (μg %)		
	No.	Mean ± SE	Range	No.	Mean ± SE	Range	No.	Mean ± SE	Range
1	11	4.0 ± 0.8	1.1 - 7.8	18	419.4 ± 46.6	128 - 797			
6	25	2.0 ± 0.3	0.3 - 7.5	26	168.7 ± 25.8	39.2 - 604			
7	22	1.6 ± 0.4	0.2 - 7.2	23	150.2 ± 21.6	10.6 - 348			
8	14	7.2 ± 1.3	1.2 - 14.2	17	787.9 ± 101.4	92.4 - 1449.6	8	23.1 ± 3.1	11.7 - 34.4
9	10	2.4 ± 0.4	0.3 - 4.1	11	281.5 ± 57.8	57.8 - 678.6	30	18.2 ± 1.5	3.2 - 37.4
10	30	2.8 ± 0.4	0.1 - 7.7	36	118.9 ± 17.2	4.0 - 397.2	20	9.6 ± 1.0	3.4 - 15.8
11	13	3.3 ± 0.6	1.0 - 9.2	18	242.5 ± 29.7	50.2 - 446.4	13	13.5 ± 1.6	3.4 - 24.4
Total	125	3.1 ± 0.3	0.1 - 14.2	149	272 ± 22.9	4.0 - 1449.6	71	15.4 ± 1.0	3.2 - 37.4

From: Galicich, Haus, Halberg, and French, 1964.

Table 2. VARIANCE SPECTRUM OF 17-HYDROXYCORTICOSTEROID CONCENTRATION (μG PER CENT) IN CANINE ADRENAL VENOUS EFFLUENT

Period (hours)	Spectral Estimate	Confidence Interval of CQ	
		0.5 Limit	0.95 Limit
24.0	1663	863	2677
24.0	1883	977	3032
12.0	1879	975	3025
8.0	1217	631	1959
6.0	614	318	988
4.8	679	353	1094
4.0	910	472	1464
3.4	751	390	1209
3.0	593	308	954

Pooled spectrum of data at 90 min intervals from 4 dogs. Total number of steroid determinations analyzed = 81; CQ = 53%; .05 Limit of CQ = 38%; 0.95 Limit of CQ = 71%; Total Variance = 9725. CQ is the circadian quotient which indicates the proportion of variance associated with the circadian rhythm. M = 8. M determines the resolving power in spectral analysis. (For details see Halberg and Panofsky (1961) Exp. Med. Surg. 19, 284, 323.) From: Galicich, Haus, Halberg, and French, 1964.

abolished not only the eosinophil rhythm but also a rhythm in blood lymphocytes (Brown and Dougherty, 1956).

The adrenal cycle appears to be an internal pacemaker of some but not all aspects of the mammalian circadian system; thus, a circadian rhythm in serum iron persists after adrenalectomy in man. The adrenal cycle is prominent under conditions which obliterate the estrus cycle, suggesting that a mammal confronted with a choice between the adrenal and the reproductive cycles chooses the former -- that is, his own survival over that of the species (Halberg and Visscher, 1952).

Circadian changes in the susceptibility of the mouse to many agents, including an adrenal inhibitor, SU-4885, can tip the scale between death and survival from this agent (Ertel, Halberg, and Ungar, 1964). In turning from the total organism to circadian rhythmic variables in blood, widely differing extents are found. Figure 8 shows, at the left, time plots of blood eosinophil counts for two groups of healthy human subjects and for a group of patients with adrenocortical insufficiency; cosinor results on these data are shown on the right. For the healthy subjects,

Table 3. VARIANCE SPECTRUM OF 17-HYDROXYCORTICOSTEROID OUTPUT (μG/MIN) IN CANINE ADRENAL VENOUS EFFLUENT

Period (hours)	Spectral Estimate	Confidence Interval of CQ	
		.05 Limit	.95 Limit
24.0	1.94	.68	3.72
24.0	2.89	1.01	5.55
12.0	2.69	.94	5.16
8.0	1.24	.43	2.38
6.0	.51	.18	.97
4.8	.13	.05	.25
4.0	.42	.15	.81
3.4	.44	.15	.84
3.0	.23	.08	.44

Pooled spectrum of data obtained at 90 min intervals from 3 dogs. Total number of values analyzed = 39; CQ = 72%; .05 Limit of CQ = 42%; .95 Limit = 100%. Total Variance = 8.5; M = 8. From: Galicich, Haus, Halberg, and French, 1964.

the cosinor objectively detects the rhythm and it also quantifies the relatively large circadian amplitude, A, and the rather consistent acrophase of the rhythm, ϕ. The eosinophil rhythm is not detected by cosinor in data from subjects with adrenocortical insufficiency. Such findings (Halberg, Visscher, Flink, Berge, and Bock, 1951; Kaine, Seltzer, and Conn, 1955) suggest that the circadian blood eosinophil rhythm of man, as well as that of the mouse (Halberg, Visscher, and Bittner, 1953; Brown and Dougherty, 1956), depends upon a functional adrenal cortex, whereas another circadian rhythm in human blood, namely that in serum iron, does persist in adrenocortical insufficiency (Howard, 1952; Halberg, Halberg, Barnum, and Bittner, 1959).

In experimental animals adrenocortical control of one or another aspect of circadian periodicity is required for mitoses in pinnal epidermis and in hepatic phospholipid labeling, as well as for blood eosinophil and lymphocyte counts. The adrenocortical activation precedes the onset of daily activity in mouse (Halberg, Peterson, and Silber, 1959) and man (Halberg, Frank, Harner, Matthews, Aaker, Graven, and Melby, 1961).

The adrenal cycle has been traced to the venous effluent of the cannulated dog adrenal; a circadian rhythm and also less prominent, yet statistically significant, ultradian changes -- with a frequency higher than one cycle in 20 hours -- are found in the 17-hydroxycorticosteroid

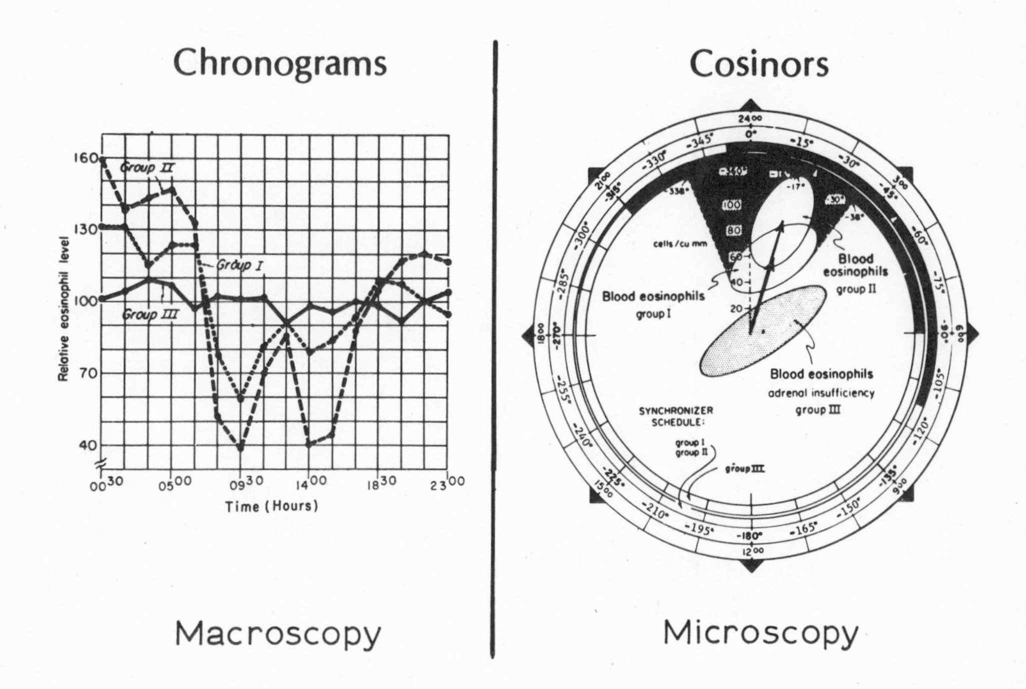

Figure 8. *Time plots of 3 sets of transverse data on relative changes in blood eosinophil counts (left), analyzed by cosinor (right). Note the flat curve for blood eosinophil counts of group III, consisting of patients with adrenal insufficiency. The corresponding error ellipse (right) overlaps the pole -- thus a rhythm is not detected. For the data on groups I and II, consisting of healthy subjects, the rhythm is detected by the relatively tight error ellipses, away from the pole. The circadian acrophase, ϕ, is the angle formed by a vector with the radius pointing to zero degrees; the ϕ values for groups I and II both on similar synchronizer schedules prior to the sampling span, are similar. From: Halberg, Visscher, Flink, Berge, and Bock, 1951.*

released from the gland (Galicich, Haus, Halberg, and French, 1964), Tables 1-3. In the mouse, circadian rhythmic changes have been mapped in cooperation with P. Albrecht, R. Silber, R. Peterson, E. Haus, and F. Ungar for the directly extracted corticosterone content of the gland (Figure 9) and for the slope of the in vitro corticosterone production

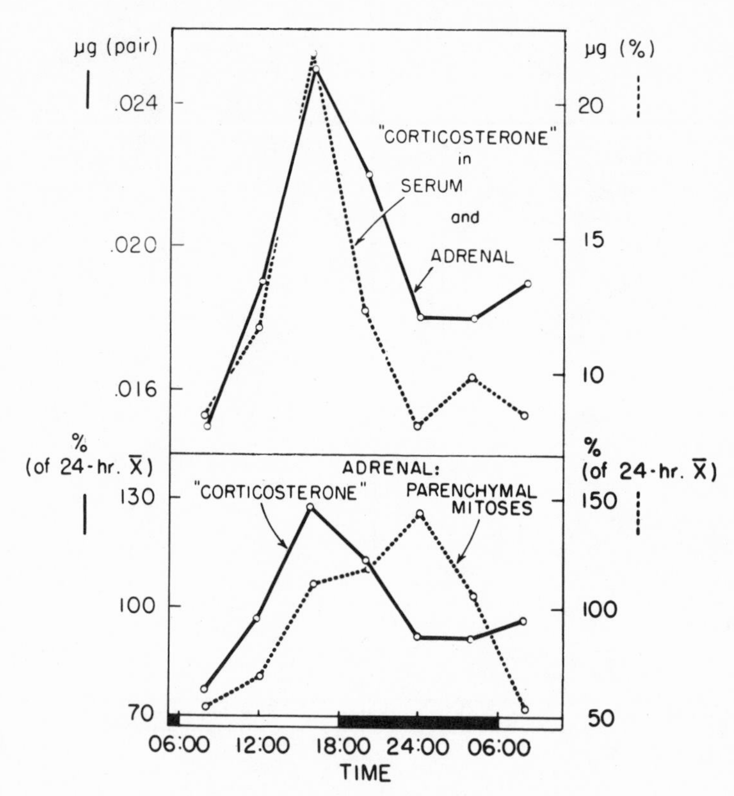

Figure 9. Circadian rhythms of corticosterone in mouse blood and adrenal and their time relation to the mitotic rhythm in glandular parenchyma. From: Halberg, Peterson, and Silber, 1959.

by the gland following the addition of graded doses of ACTH to the incubation fluid (Figure 10) and for pituitary adrenocorticotropic activity (Figure 11) as well as for hypothalamic CRF (Ungar and Halberg, 1962, 1963; Halberg, 1964). Even the respiration of the hamster adrenal in organ culture is reportedly circadian rhythmic (Andrews and Folk, 1964) as is corticosterone production (Andrews and Shiotsuka, 1974).

A circadian reactivity rhythm of the mouse adrenal to ACTH also can be demonstrated in vivo (Haus and Halberg, 1962) with a timing corresponding to that found in vitro. In vivo, the adrenal response to

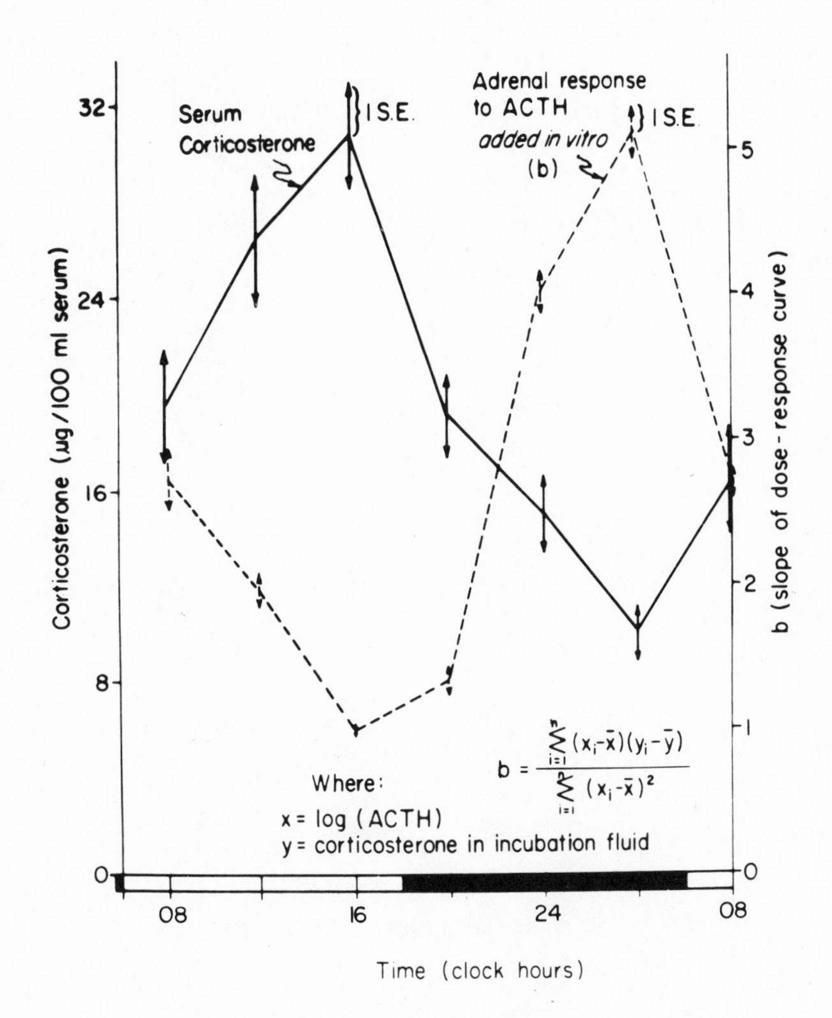

$$b = \frac{\sum_{i=1}^{n}(x_i-\bar{x})(y_i-\bar{y})}{\sum_{i=1}^{n}(x_i-\bar{x})^2}$$

Figure 10. *Circadian periodic response of mouse adrenals to ACTH added in vitro. Total of seven-hundred C-mouse adrenals incubated. Time relations of circadian rhythms in serum corticosterone (solid line, mean of 12 pools each from 5 mice per time point, total of 420 C-mice), and in adrenal responsivity to ACTH in vitro (broken line, slope of log dose-response relation of quartered adrenals to ACTH added in vitro). From: Haus and Halberg, 1962; Haus, Halberg, Kühl, and Lakatua, 1974.*

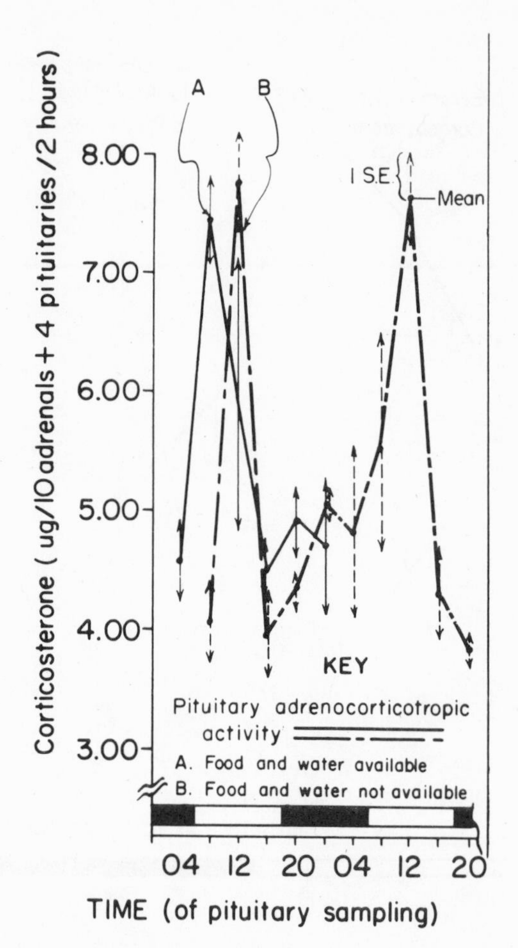

Figure 11. Demonstrates prominent rhythms in pituitary adrenocorticotropic activity, both in the presence and absence of food and water. Although many rhythms persist during starvation and dehydration until death, some of these same rhythms have been demonstrated to be amenable to phase-shifting by manipulation of mealtime. Moreover, mealtime has proved to be a determinant of internal timing within the circadian system and has been documented under special conditions to tip the scale between death and survival. From: Halberg, Galicich, Ungar, and French, 1965.

saline also exhibits a circadian rhythm with a large reproducible timing and high statistical significance (Haus and Halberg, 1962); the time of maximal in vivo response to ACTH differs drastically from the timing of the crest in reactivity to another stimulus applied to the adrenal cortex, such as saline. The stability of the circadian rhythm in the more or less spontaneous activity of the rodent's adrenal cortex and this gland's reactivity to ACTH is remarkable.

The adrenal cycle's ϕ is adaptable, within limits, to modifications of routine. An abrupt change in the so-called environmental synchronizer, such as a displacement along the 24-hour scale of the temporal location of alternating 12-hour spans of light and darkness, is followed by a gradual rather than sudden change in ϕ of the circadian rhythms in blood eosinophil counts and serum corticosterone (Halberg, Visscher, and Bittner, 1953; Halberg, Barnum, Silber, and Bittner, 1958). Moreover, one can shift by meal-timing in the mouse (though not in man), the timing of rhythms in serum corticosterone (Nelson, Halberg, and Scheving, unpublished), and in blood eosinophils (Scheving, Halberg, Pauly, Burns, Tsai, and Betterton, 1973). Some of the effects of the lighting regimen are mediated by the eyes (Figure 3); after bilateral optic enucleation, the synchronization of circadian rhythms with the lighting cycle is lost. At three weeks following the blinding of inbred C-mice, a serum corticosterone rhythm is grossly in antiphase when compared in terms of its timing with the rhythm of concomitantly studied sham-operated mice. Blinding results in the loss of external synchronization, but the rhythm continues to occur with a roughly unaltered amplitude. Moreover, the rhythm assumes a new frequency which varies slightly but with statistical significance among individual animals, say from 23.3 to 23.7 hours, while it differs again with statistical significance, from a ϕ equal to 24 hours as well. Such persisting frequencies, for which environmental counterparts are not known, indicate that the environmental synchronizing information transmitted by the eyes is not essential for the maintenance of circadian rhythmicity in body temperature of mice. The eyes also were dispensable for the maintenance of time relations among certain circadian rhythms. Table 4 shows that the internal timing in relation to the body temperature rhythm of the rhythms in serum corticosterone and in liver glycogen is clearly maintained in male as well as in female C-mice at three weeks after blinding -- a time point chosen for this spot-check on the basis of analyses in Figure 3. For C-mice of both sexes there is thus a state of external circadian desynchronization following blinding, when, on the average only, certain functions of the mouse run on a 23.4 or 23.5 hour cycle. In the face of this external desynchronization, there can persist an internal circadian synchronization in some circadian rhythmic physiologic variables. By the same token, in human beings studied in caves under conditions of isolation from time cues for spans of several months, certain functions continue to exhibit some prominent circadian rhythms (Siffre, Reinberg, Halberg, Ghata, Perdriel, and Slind, 1966), whereas sleep-wakefulness in turn may exhibit infradian rhythmic components ($\tau > 28$ hours) that, as in two subjects, were slightly more prominent than the circadian one.

Table 4. *INTERNAL TIMING OF TWO CIRCADIAN BIOCHEMICAL RHYTHMS IN RELATION TO THAT IN RECTAL TEMPERATURE IN MATURE MALE (M) OR FEMALE (F) INBRED C-MICE*

Sex	τ* hours	Phase, ϕ (.95 confidence arc) expressed as delay			or advance
		Rectal temperature	Liver glycogen	Serum corticosterone	
		Sham-operation: 24-hour synchronized rhythms			
M	24.0	0 (-325° to -36°)	- 81° (- 72° to - 90°)	-265° (-237° to -293°)	+95°
F	24.0	0 (-343° to -17°)	- 96° (- 85° to -108°)	-267° (-230° to -304°)	+93°
		Blinding: externally desyncrhonized rhythms			
M	23.4	0 (-345° to -15°)	-122° (- 84° to -161°)	-305° (-240° to - 11°)	+55°
F	23.5	0 (-352° to - 8°)	-131° (-117° to -144°)	-275° (-261° to -288°)	+85°

τ = 360°; rounded numbers; ϕ in relation to 00⁰⁰ on December 31, 1899; ϕ can be converted to local clock-time only in the case of a 24-hour τ (360° = 24 hours). From: Haus, Lakatua, and Halberg, 1967.

VIII. WIDE DOMAIN OF BIOLOGIC RHYTHM FREQUENCIES

Today several important points can be made in light of amply documented facts (Scheving, Halberg, and Pauly, 1974). First, rhythms are so general as to constitute a fundamental property of most living matter. Their degree of generality is reflected in the wide domain of frequencies encountered in their recurrence. Two heartbeats can be separated by less than a second -- they are part of a short period (high-frequency) rhythm. Two menstruations can be separated by more than a month -- they constitute an expression of the long period (low-frequency) rhythm displayed by the human ovary, expressed in menstruation. Both heart rate and menstruation constitute components in a wider spectrum of physiologic rhythms. The electroencephalogram, representing electrical activity of the brain, shows frequencies near one cycle per second and up to thirty times higher. The urinary excretion of norepinephrine from the adrenal glands reveals a spectrum of rhythms, including a circadian and a circannual component superimposed upon a decrease in amplitude with advancing age (Descovich, Montalbetti, Kühl, Rimondi, and Halberg, 1973).

IX. GRADUAL AND POLAR RHYTHM ADJUSTMENT

Rhythms adjust their timing after individuals cross several time zones by jet or change work schedules without geographic displacement. Such adjustment is gradual and polar (directed); it occurs at differing rates as a function of whether a schedule is advanced (e.g., after a flight from west to east) or delayed (e.g., after a flight from east to west). The resulting transient desynchronization, denoted as transmeridian dyschronism, may contribute the proverbial straw to break the camel's back. Performance decrement after certain transmeridian flights can, if any, be slight; yet the net result is not negligible when peak "output" in extremely athletic or other talented or politically important individuals is the case in point, or when the overall sometimes critical performance of large numbers of individuals (troops) or the survival of debilitated patients is at stake.

X. RHYTHMS RELEVANT TO HEALTH CARE

The key point in this discussion is the importance of rhythms under controlled laboratory conditions; the predictably changing state of organism's rhythms tips the scale between death and survival from a variety of potentially harmful agents. Quite apart from what we have learned about susceptibility to ethanol (Halberg, 1960; Haus and Halberg, 1959), a fixed dose of a drug now used in treating heart disease (Halberg, 1953) or cancer (Cardoso, Scheving, and Halberg, 1970; Haus, Halberg, Scheving, Cardoso, Kühl, Sothern, Shiotsuka, Hwang, and Pauly, 1972; Halberg, Haus, Cardoso, Scheving, Kühl, Shiotsuka, Rosene, Pauly, Runge, Spalding, Lee, and Good, 1973) or of a poison derived from bacteria (Halberg, Johnson, Brown, and Bittner, 1960) or even of noise in susceptible animals (Halberg, Jacobson, Wadsworth, and Bittner, 1958) will kill or not, de-

pending on the stage of the experimental animals' rhythms. Circadian and circannual susceptibility rhythms in mice or rats are relevant to changes in human disease and death (Smolensky, Halberg, and Sargent, 1972; Aycock, Lutman, and Foley, 1945; Aycock, Foley, and Hendrie, 1946; Frost and Gover, 1932; Gafafer, 1931; Lillie, Dyer, Armstrong, and Pasternack, 1937; Pearce, Brown, and Van Allen, 1924; Pritchett, 1925; Webster, 1927; Wilson, 1930). Statistically significant differences in sickness or in mortality from certain diseases as a function of clock-hour or season have long been confirmed but one could not know from such statistics whether internal factors contributed in any way to these variations in mortality. These variations can be viewed in conjunction with controlled susceptibility studies on man; and with the added background of investigations on experimental animals, the critical importance of innate cycles in mechanisms of resistance becomes readily apparent. We now can raise questions concerning the relative contributions of purely internal and purely external causes of rhythms and perhaps find that some rhythms can be manipulated to improve health and lengthen life.

Rhythms deserve attention because they are basic, relevant, and ever-present phenomena in human beings and in most, if not all, other forms of life -- plants as well as animals.

The concrete science which studies time characteristics in life forms -- chronobiology -- should be incorporated into the school curriculum at various levels. Information on rhythms can be taught in conjunction with the self-measurement of body functions throughout high school, and even earlier, as part of the existing science curriculum. Several benefits can thereby be derived at negligible cost. Instead of relying exclusively on complex man-made instruments and on life forms other than human beings, one can study important biologic concepts with one's own body as a continuously and freely available remarkable "instrument." Furthermore, a data base thus gained can be utilized for immediate preventive health care and also for later diagnostic and curative action by the physician -- quite apart from its usefulness in the educative process. The health performance data collected by self-measurement, or by automatic recording instruments, can be summarized in a variety of chronobiologic displays. The results of analyses can be charted as an individual data base which might eventually be summarized on a health form combined perhaps with blood group and other information on a social security card or driver's license (Halberg, 1973).

XI. RHYTHMS IN PREVENTIVE MEDICINE

Information on blood pressure, heart rate, and body temperature collected while the subject is in apparent health will be particularly helpful to the family physician because it provides information on his patient that can no longer be secured once disease has set in. Such data can be obtained not only by the student but also by parents, relatives, and friends motivated by enthusiastic disciples to carry out self-measurements. If contacted via other health care or screening channels, these same individuals would be less likely to take time to attend special classes.

The World Health Organization has declared high blood pressure "a widespread epidemic" and has called for physicians and the public to be aware of and treat its dangers. Only a small fraction of the men and women who suffer from hypertension know about it, and an even smaller fraction receive correct or adequate treatment. Hence, education and implementation of self-measurement procedures should receive top priority.

It is easy to learn the simple procedures of taking and recording physiologic and psychologic measurements. It may not be too taxing to continue such measurements over a sufficiently long time span to gain information concerning individualized "usual range" of values for the subject. In order to take self-measurements, the participant needs proper yet eventually inexpensive (if mass-produced) instruments and a knowledge of how to use them. Observations can be made on a schedule involving regular hours of sleep and eating. Cardiovascular and psychomotor performance can be gauged by systolic and diastolic blood pressure, pulse, grip strength, and eye-hand coordination among others -- all readily self-measured. Oral temperature also should be taken and mood and vigor rated, e.g., on a seven-point scale. For assessing subjective "tempo," one minute can be estimated by counting from 1 to 60 and recording the time actually elapsed with a stopwatch. Peak expiratory flow (how hard one can blow) can be measured to assess an aspect of lung function; this same variable in sensitive subjects such as patients with so-called extrinsic asthma will change markedly under some conditions of air pollution and can thus constitute a biologic warning indicator (Reinberg, Gervais, Halberg, and Halberg, 1971).

XII. CHRONOTHERAPY

The exploitation of information about rhythms has also begun in the clinic; thus when a given prominent hormonal rhythm is absent, as in the case of Addison's disease, substitution treatment can be timed not only to reproduce the periodicity but also to locate optimal performance, such as grip strength, according to the requirements (e.g., work times) of the patient (Reinberg, Ghata, Halberg, Apfelbaum, Gervais, Boudon, Abulker, and Dupont, 1971).

Drug testing is rendered more efficient when undue variability is reduced by evaluating rhythms and carrying out work in defined stages of predictable cycles. As an optimum achieved thus far, rhythm assessment allows timing according to predictable changes that improve tolerance of a widely used carcinostatic drug (Haus, Halberg, Scheving, Cardoso, Kühl, Sothern, Shiotsuka, Hwang, and Pauly, 1972; Halberg, Haus, Cardoso, Scheving, Kühl, Shiotsuka, Rosene, Pauly, Runge, Spalding, Lee, and Good, 1973).

With respect to host tolerance, the implication that sinusoidal dosage schedules may markedly improve the therapeutic index (i.e., decrease the toxicity relative to the effectiveness [curative action]) of an anti-metabolite, ara-C, and perhaps that of many other drugs, at the bedside, is inescapable. The increase in tolerance already effectively achieved is not a trivial one; it could thus represent definitively the difference between success and failure in therapeutic application.

Finally, focus upon the tumor's possible rhythms in addition to those of the host is warranted.

A chronotherapeutic index (CTI) was defined as CTI = PST x TVC, where PST = individual's percent survival time relative to overall mean (=100%) of all treated individuals irrespective of treatment time, and TVC = individual's extrapolated 47-hour post-treatment tumor volume change: a) relative to individual's extrapolated 1-hour pre-treatment tumor volume, and b) expressed as ratio a/b. Results thus analyzed show for mice in light from 06^{00} to 18^{00}, alternating with darkness, the highest CTI (=122%) at 22^{00}, the second highest CTI (=104%) at 02^{00}, and the lowest CTI (=8%) at 18^{00}. A 24-hour cosine model fitted by least squares showed statistical significance for the original mean survival times, for survival times expressed as percentage of overall mean, and for CTI (Halberg, Haus, Cardoso, Scheving, Kühl, Shiotsuka, Rosene, Pauly, Runge, Spalding, Lee, and Good, 1973).

REFERENCES

Andrews, R. V. (1968). Temporal secretory responses of cultured hamster adrenals. Comp. Biochem. Physiol. 26, 179.

Andrews, R. V. and Folk, G. E., Jr. (1964). Circadian metabolic patterns in cultured hamster adrenal glands. Comp. Biochem. Physiol. 11, 393.

Andrews, R. V. and Shiotsuka, R. (1974). In vitro adrenal studies in relation to cyclic reproductive success. In: *Biorhythms and Human Reproduction - Proceedings of the International Institute for the Study of Human Reproduction* (Ferin, M., Halberg, F., Richart, R., and Vande Wiele, R., eds.), pp. 591-605, Wiley, New York.

Aschoff, J. (1960). Exogenous and endogenous components in circadian rhythms. Cold Spring Harbor Symp. Quant. Biol. 25, 11-28.

Aycock, W. L., Foley, G. E., and Hendrie, K. H. (1946). The epidemiologic significance of amplitudes of seasonal fluctuation in infectious disease. Am. J. Med. Sci. 211, 709.

Aycock, W. L., Lutman, G. E., and Foley, G. E. (1945). Seasonal prevalence as a principle in epidemiology. Am. J. Med. Sci. 209, 395.

Brown, H. E. and Dougherty, T. F. (1956). The diurnal variation of blood leucocytes in normal and adrenalectomized mice. Endocrinology 58, 365.

Cardoso, S. S., Scheving, L. E., and Halberg, F. (1970). Mortality of mice as influenced by the hour of the day of drug (ara-C) administration. Pharmacologist 12, 302.

Descovich, G. C., Montalbetti, N., Kühl, J. F. W., Rimondi, S., and Halberg, F. (1973). Circadian as well as circannual in-phase synchronization of urinary epinephrine (E) and norepinephrine (NE) and acrophase-difference of E or NE with NER = NE/(NE+E) in mature and presumably health human beings. Int. J. Chronobiol. 1, 324.

Einstein, A. (1905). Zur electrodynamik bewegter Körper. Ann. Phys. (Leipzig) 322, 891-921.

Einstein, A. (1920). *Relativity: The special and general theory*, Methuen, London.
Einstein, A. (1922). *Sidelights on relativity*, Methuen, London.
Ertel, R. J., Halberg, F., and Ungar, F. (1964). Circadian system phase-dependent toxicity and other effects of methopyrapone (SU-4885) in mice. J. Pharmacol. Exp. Ther. 146, 395-399.
Frost, W. H. and Gover, M. (1932). The incidence and time distribution of common colds in several groups kept under continuous observation. Weekly Pub. Health Rep. 47, 1815.
Gafafer, W. M. (1931). Upper respiratory disease (common cold) and the weather. Am. J. Hyg. 13, 771.
Galicich, J. H., Haus, E., Halberg, F., and French, L. A. (1964). Variance spectra of corticosteroid in adrenal venous effluent of anesthetized dogs. Ann. N.Y. Acad. Sci. 117, 281-291.
Hafele, J. C. and Keating, R. E. (1972). Around-the-World-Atomic-Clocks: Observed relativisitc time gains. Science 177, 166.
Halberg, F. (1953). Some physiological and clinical aspects of 24-hour periodicity. Lancet 73, 20-32.
Halberg, F. (1954). Beobachtungen über 24 Stunden-Periodik in standardisierter Versuchsanordnung vor und nach Epinephrektomie und bilateraler optischer Enukleation. Ber. Ges. Physiol. 162, 354-355.
Halberg, F. (1960). Temporal coordination of physiologic function. Cold Spring Harbor Symp. Quant. Biol. 25, 289-310.
Halberg, F. (1961). Circadian aspects of mitosis and metabolism. Rep. Ross Conf. Pediatr. Res. 39, 41-44.
Halberg, F. (1965). Organisms as circadian systems; temporal analysis of their physiologic and pathologic responses, including injury and death. In: *Symposium on Medical Aspects of Stress in the Military Climate, Proceedings*, pp. 1-36, Walter Reed Army Institute of Research, Washington.
Halberg, F. (1968). Physiologic considerations underlying rhythmometry, with special reference to emotional illness. In: *Biological Cycles and Psychiatry, Symposium Bel-Air III* (de Ajuriaguerra, J., ed.), pp. 73-126, Masson, Geneva.
Halberg, F. (1969). Chronobiology. Annu. Rev. Physiol. 31, 675-725.
Halberg, F. (1970). Body temperature, circadian rhythms and the eye. In: *La Photoregulation de la Reproduction chez les Oiseaux et les Mammiferes* (Benoit, J. and Assenmacher, I., eds.), pp. 497-528, Centre National de la Recherche Scientifique, Paris.
Halberg, F. (1973). Chronobiology and its promise for health care and environmental integrity. Int. J. Chronobiol. 1, 10-14.
Halberg, F., Barnum, C. P., Silber, R. H., and Bittner, J. J. (1958). 24-hour rhythms at several levels of integration in mice on different lighting regimens. Proc. Soc. Exp. Biol. Med. 97, 897-900.
Halberg, F., Engeli, M., Hamburger, C., and Hillman, D. (1965). Spectral resolution of low-frequency, small-amplitude rhythms in excreted ketosteroid; probable androgen-induced circaseptan desynchronization. Acta Endocrinol. (Suppl.) 103, 54.
Halberg, F., Frank, G., Harner, R., Matthews, J., Aaker, H., Gravem, H., and Melby, J. (1961). The adrenal cycle in men on different schedules of motor and mental activitiy. Experientia 17, 282.

Halberg, F., Galicich, J. H., Ungar, F., and French, L. A. (1965). Circadian rhythmic pituitary adrenocorticotropic activity, rectal temperature and pinnal mitosis of starving, dehydrated C-mice. Proc. Soc. Exp. Biol. Med. 118, 414-419.

Halberg, F., Halberg, E., Barnum, C. P., and Bittner, J. J. (1959). Physiologic 24-hour periodicity in human beings and mice, the lighting regimen and daily routine. In: *Photoperiodism and Related Phenomena in Plants and Animals* (Withrow, R. B. ed.), pp. 803-878, Am. Assoc. Adv. Sci., Washington.

Halberg, F., Halberg, J., Halberg, F., and Halberg, E. (1973). Reading, 'riting, 'rithmetic ... and rhythms -- a new "relevant" "R" in the educative process. Perspect. Biol. Med. 17, 128-141.

Halberg, F., Haus, E., Cardoso, S. S., Scheving, L. E., Kühl, J. F. W., Shiotsuka, R., Rosene, G., Pauly, J. E., Runge, W., Spalding, J. F., Lee, J. K., and Good, R. A. (1973). Toward a chronotherapy of neoplasia: tolerance of treatment depends upon host rhythms. Experientia 29, 909-934.

Halberg, F., Jacobson, E., Wadsworth, G., and Bittner, J. J. (1958). Audiogenic abnormality spectra, 24-hour periodicity and lighting. Science 128, 657-658.

Halberg, F., Johnson, E. A., Brown, B. W., and Bittner, J. J. (1960). Susceptibility rhythm to E. coli endotoxin and bioassay. Proc. Soc. Exp. Biol. Med. 103, 142-144.

Halberg, F., Katinas, G. S., Chiba, Y., Garcia-Sainz, M., Kovats, T. G., Kunkel, H., Montalbetti, N., Reinberg, A., Scharf, R., and Simpson, H. (1973). Chronobiologic glossary of the International Society for the Study of Biological Rhythms. Inter. J. Chronobiol. 1, 31-63

Halberg, F., Loewenson, R., Winter, F., Bearman, J., and Adkins, J. (1960). Physiologic circadian systems (differences in period of circadian rhythms or in their component frequencies; some methodologic implications to biology and medicine). Minn. Acad. Sci. 28, 53-57.

Halberg, F., Nelson, W., Runge, W. J., Schmitt, O. H., Pitts, G. C., Tremor, J., and Reynolds, O. E. (1971). Plans for orbital study of rat biorhythms. Results of interest beyond the biosatellite program. Space Life Sci. 2, 437-471

Halberg, F., Peterson, R. E., and Silber, R. H. (1959). Phase relations of 24-hour periodicities in blood corticosterone, mitoses in cortical adrenal parenchyma and total body activity. Endocrinology 64, 222-230.

Halberg, F. and Reinberg, A. (1967). Rythmes circadiens et rythmes de basses fréquences en physiologie humaine. J. Physiol. 59, 117-200.

Halberg, F., Reinberg, A., Haus, E., Ghata, J., and Siffre, M. (1970). Human biological rhythms during and after several months of isolation underground in natural caves. Natl. Speleol. Soc. Bull. 32, 89-115.

Halberg, F. and Simpson, H. (1967). Circadian acrophases of human 17-hydroxycorticosteroid excretion referred to midsleep rather than midnight. Hum. Biol. 39, 405-413.

Halberg, F. and Visscher, M. B. (1952). Effect of light and of availability of food upon the 24-hour rhythm in number of circulating eosinophils in mice. Am. J. Physiol. 171, 732.

Halberg, F., Visscher, M. B., and Bittner, J. J. (1953). Eosinophil rhythm in mice: Range of occurrence; effects of illumination, feeding, and adrenalectomy. Am. J. Physiol. 174, 313-315.

Halberg, F., Visscher, M. B., Flink, E. B., Berge, K., and Bock, R. (1951). Diurnal rhythmic changes in blood eosinophil levels in health and in certain diseases. Lancet 71, 312-319.

Halberg, F. and Visscher, M. B. (1952). A difference between the effects of dietary calorie restriction on the estrus cycle and on the 24-hour adrenal cortical cycle in rodents. Endocrinology 51, 329-335.

Haus, E., Halberg, F., Kühl, J. F. W., and Lakatua, D. J. (1974). Chronopharmacology in animals. In: *Capri Symposium* (In Press).

Haus, E. and Halberg, F. (1962). Der circadiane Adrenalzyklus und seine Bedeutung für die Reaktionsbereitschaft der Nebennierenrinde. Wien. Z. Inn. Med. 8, 361-370.

Haus, E., Lakatua, D., and Halberg, F. (1967). The internal timing of several circadian rhythms in the blinded mouse. Exp. Med. Surg. 25, 7-45.

Haus, E. (1964). Periodicity in response and susceptibility to environmental stimuli. Ann. N.Y. Acad. Sci. 117, 292-315.

Haus, E. and Halberg, F. (1959). 24-hour rhythm in susceptibility of C-mice to a toxic dose of ethanol. J. Appl. Physiol. 14, 878-880.

Haus, E. and Halberg, F. (1962). Interactions of a chemical carcinogen with neuroendocrine factors in mouse breast cancer. Experientia 18, 340-341.

Haus, E., Halberg, F., Scheving, L., Cardoso, S., Kühl, J., Sothern, R., Shiotsuka, R., Hwang, D. S., and Pauly, J. E. (1972). Increased tolerance of leukemic mice to arabinosyl cytosine given on a schedule adjusted-to circadian system. Science 177, 80-82.

Hellbrügge, Th. (1960). The development of circadian rhythms in infants. Cold Spring Harbor Symp. Quant. Biol. 25, 311-324.

Howard, R. B. (1952). *Studies on the Metabolism of Iron,* Ph.D. Thesis, University of Minnesota, Minneapolis.

Kaine, H. D., Seltzer, H. S., and Conn, J. W. (1955). Mechanisms of diurnal eosinophil rhythm in man. J. Lab. Clin. Med. 45, 247.

Lillie, R. D., Dyer, R. E., Armstrong, C., and Pasternack, J. G. (1937). Seasonal variation in intensity of brain reaction of St. Louis encephalitis in mice and of endemic typhus in guinea pigs. Public Health Rep. 52, 1805.

Mills, J. N. (1967). Circadian rhythms and shift workers. Trans. Soc. Occup. Med. 17, 5-7.

Pearce, L., Brown, W. H., and Van Allen, C. M. (1924). Studies based on a malignant tumor of the rabbit. IV. Variations in growth and malignancy of transplanted tumors. Part 2: Factors influencing the results of serial transplantation. J. Exp. Med. 40, 603.

Pittendrigh, C. S. (1960). Circadian rhythms and the circadian organization of living systems. Cold Spring Harbor Symp. Quant. Biol. 25, 159-184.

Pritchett, I. W. (1925). Microbic virulence and host susceptibility in paratyphoid -- enteritidis infection of white mice. VII. Seasonal variation in the susceptibility of different strains of mice to per os infection with the Type II bacillus of mouse typhoid. J. Exp. Med. 41, 209.

Reimann, H. (1963). *Periodic Diseases*, Davis, Philadelphia.

Reinberg, A., Gervais, P., Halberg, F., and Halberg, F. (1971). Trisentinel monitoring of air pollution by autorhythmometry of peak expiratory flow. In: *Proceedings of the Second International Clean Air Congress* (Englund, H. M. and Berry, W. T., eds.), pp. 217-220, Academic, New York.

Reinberg, A., Ghata, J., Halberg, F., Apfelbaum, M., Gervais, P., Boudon, P., Abulker, C., and Dupont, J. (1971). Distribution temporelle du traitement de l'insuffisance corticosurrenaliene -- essai de chronotherapeutique. Ann. Endocrinol. 32, 566-573.

Rummel, J. A., Lee, J. K., and Halberg, F. (In Press). Combined linear-non-linear chronobiologic windows by least squares resolve neighboring components in a physiologic rhythm spectrum. In: *Biorhythms and Human Reproduction - Proceedings of the International Institute for the Study of Human Reproduction* (Ferin, M., Halberg, F., Richart, R., and Vande Wiele, R., eds.), pp. 53-82, Wiley, New York.

Santorio, S. (1957). *De Statica Medicina*, Vlaco, Hague.

Scheving, L. E., Halberg, F., and Pauly, J. E. (eds.) (1974). *Chronobiology - Proceedings of the International Society for the Study of Biological Rhythms*, Igaku Shoin, Ltd., Tokyo.

Scheving, L., Halberg, F., Pauly, J. E., Burns, E. R., Tsai, S., and Betterton, H. (1973). Lighting regimen dominates over interacting meal schedules and synchronizes mitotic rhythm in mouse corneal epithelium. Anat. Rec. (In Press).

Shiotsuka, R., Jovonovich, J., and Jovonovich, J. (1974). Circadian and ultradian rhythms in adrenal organ cultures. In: *Capri Symposium* (In Press).

Siffre, M., Reinberg, A., Halberg, F., Ghata, J., Perdriel, G., and Slind, R. (1966). L'isolement souterrain prolonge. Etude de deux sujets adultes sains avant, pendant et apres cet isolement. Presse Med. 74, 915-919.

Simpson, H. W., Gjessing, L., Fleck, A., Kühl, J., and Halberg, F. (1974). Phase analysis of the somatic and mental variables in Gjessing's case 2484 or intermittent catatonia. In: *Chronobiology - Proceedings of the International Society for the Study of Biological Rhythms* (Scheving, L. E., Halberg, F., and Pauly, J. E., eds.), pp. 535-539, Igaku Shoin, Ltd., Tokyo.

Smolensky, M., Halberg, F., and Sargent, F. (1972). Chronobiology of the life sequence. In: *Advances in Climatic Physiology* (Itoh, S., Ogata, K., and Yoshimura, H., eds.), pp. 281-318, Igaku Shoin, Ltd., Tokyo.

Terrell, J. (1972). The clock "paradox" -- majority view. Phys. Today 25, 9.

Ungar, F. and Halberg, F. (1962). Circadian rhythm in the in vitro response of mouse adrenal to adrenocorticotropic hormone. Science 137, 1058.
Ungar, F. and Halberg, F. (1963). In vitro demonstration of circadian rhythm in adrenocorticotropic activity of C-mouse hypophysis. Experientia 19, 158.
Webster, L. T. (1927). Epidemiologic studies on respiratory infection in the rabbit. IX. The spread of Bacterium lepisepticum infection at a rabbit farm in New York City. J. Exp. Med. 45, 529-551.
Wilson, G. S. (1930). Transient fluctuations in the resistance of mice to infection with B. aertryche. J. Hyg. 30, 196.

DISCUSSION AFTER DR. HALBERG'S PAPER

Dr. Krieger

Would you like to speculate on what you said was probably one of the most exciting findings, namely, the mechanism of shifting the periodicity by altered eating cycles? I think there is no doubt that this does exist. We'll show a little bit of our own data tomorrow, and I think there are also data indicating that not only shifting of food intake, but just mere shifting of water intake will shift the periodicity. Having made these observations, would you like to speculate as to what the mechanism would be in the face of normal light-dark cycle?

Dr. Halberg

We have not studied separately any effects from the timing of access to water in competition with effects from restricted access to food at different times. In cooperation with several investigators (Halberg et al., 1953; Nelson et al., 1973; Nelson et al., 1973; Nelson et al., submitted for publication; Pauly et al., submitted for publication; Pauly et al., 1973; Halberg et al., 1973; Stupfel et al., 1973a, 1973b), we have manipulated for rodents the timing of simultaneous access to both food and water, thereby shifting the very rhythm in serum corticosterone that persists so clearly in the absence of any and all food and water intake (Galicich et al., 1963; Halberg et al., 1965). I am looking forward to seeing your data on what happens if you manipulate only access to water. Moreover, in our work we have not divorced any effects related to the timing of meals from those associated with the timing of activity. This topic, investigated earlier by Bolles and Duncan (1969) deserves further scrutiny in both man and rodent.

Synchronization by social factors, actually regulating meals and activities, may indeed underlie what has been referred to since 1957 as a socio-ecologic synchronization (Halberg et al., 1959). Social factors come to mind when circadian rhythms remain 24-hour synchronized presumably by the social routine as shown by Levine et al. (1973) for a bilateral retinoblastoma studied before and after removal of both eyes.

The timing of food and water intake may not play the sole critical role in the synchronization of this child deprived suddenly of both eyes, but rather the overall hospital or home routine might be involved. Both periodic food intake, as such, and gross motor activity were somewhat controlled in another case studied by Levine et al. (1967). A child who came to the hospital for surgery of the upper lip failed to recover from anesthesia and exhibited a non-24-hour circadian period in blood pressure until the day when physical therapy was started at 10^{00} (and was continued each day at the same time thereafter). From that day on, a 24-hour synchronized rhythm was seen. In this child, the rubdown by a nurse became the dominant synchronizer of a circadian rhythm.

These two clinical cases, namely a child deprived of its eyes and another child unintentionally deprived of its consciousness, indicate that circadian synchronization by presumably complex factors is possible after eye removal and even in the absence of a functional nervous system, as in this case of human coma.

More critical studies have been possible in the same connection on experimental animals. Quite a few years ago in our laboratory at Minnesota, Galicich et al. (1965) investigated the effect upon rhythms of step-wise brain ablation. They removed first the cortex, then the thalamus, thereafter the hypothalamus, leaving a pituitary island which was then also removed so that eventually they dealt with a suprapontine brain ablation. The major findings were that at least for one complete cycle following operation, the rhythmicity of two variables, serum corticosterone and body temperature, continued. However, post-operatively the internal timing of these two rhythms had changed time relations. Before brain removal, the corticosterone rhythm led that of body temperature. After brain ablation, the temperature rhythm was leading.

From the clinical cases and basic work, one can indeed glance back at a 1958 model of a network of rhythms, elaborating on the relative (dominant or secondary) roles of different synchronizers under different conditions with respect to a few body functions. In keeping with that empirical model of 1958 we can amplify on the role of the brain in monitoring internal timing of many more circadian rhythmic body functions.

Recently we have learned not only that many and different body functions are quite differently affected by the same synchronizing schedule in the same organism when light-dark schedules are altered and meal times also are changed, but available evidence also demonstrates that under different conditions of access to food we deal with a dramatically different organism in terms of circadian system structure. Indeed, the feeding-time determined difference is of such an extent that under special conditions, survival and death can be made dependent upon the timing of access to food (Nelson et al., 1973).

What seems yet more important, we might have a different behavioral and biochemical food utilization in different circadian systems. In any event, the mouse demonstrates a statistically significantly lesser weight gain when four hours of access to food are allowed early in the activity span (in the early dark span) rather than early in the rest span (in the early light span). If one compares such results with findings on young human adults living on exactly 2000 calories, one should eat in the evening if one wishes to gain weight and conversely in the morning should one desire to lose weight (other things being as comparable as possible). This sort of "common knowledge" has not heretofore been fully documented in quantitative terms. Some fledgling human experimentation in this direction has been completed in Minnesota.

Dr. Ramaley

Do all things that cause the synchronization of rhythms such as temperature change have the same penetrability; that is, do they alter the phase quickly or slowly? You mentioned that a child in coma who began to receive physical therapy began to show a synchronization of rhythms on that same day. I've seen similar problems in animal work. For instance, just entering the animal room twice during the day, produced a shift in the peak of the adrenocortical rhythms to 4 A.M. (Ramaley, 1974). So it's obvious that some of these rhythms at least can be shifted very rapidly. My second question relates to the problem of choosing a reliable phase indicator in rhythm studies. If you are studying several rhythms, what do you choose as a reference point? You mentioned photoperiod and the sleep cycle. How can you decide what reference is best to use?

Dr. Halberg

If you study rhythm shifting for clinical purposes -- suddenly, instead of going to bed at 10 P.M. you stay up until 10 A.M. the following day and thereafter you sleep by day -- you find (a) that rhythm-shifts usually are gradual, and (b) that as a rule there are very great differences in rate of rhythm shifting, not only as a function of whether (1) the adjustment involves an advance or a delay of the rhythm (e.g., change comparable to that required after a flight from west to east or east to west, respectively) but also as a function of (2) the variable involved. For instance, in a study on five clinically healthy human beings after a flight from Minnesota to Japan (or its simulation), the urinary rhythms in calcium, sodium, and potassium excretion may already be rather well adjusted when the rhythm in 17-ketosteroids or corticoids as yet is not fully shifted. There are several new very exciting findings in connection with rhythm-shifting as a function of genetics and age. Yunis et al. (1973) cooperated in a study comparing "strong" mice (CBA) with "weak" ones (NZB), those genetically long lived being regarded as the strong ones, living for up to three or more years, whereas the weak ones die within a year and a half or thereabouts. We raised the question: Are there differences in shift-time of body temperature between the strong ones and the weak ones and also between young mice and old, whether strong or weak. Older mice (presumably "weaker" than strong ones) shifted more slowly. However, in terms of genetics, it was just the other way around. The strong mice shifted more slowly, a casual finding awaiting corroboration in a larger systemic sample (Table 1).

The second problem revolving around a reliable orthophase (right time) indicator constitutes a critical question for chronotherapy.

Table 1. CUMULATIVE EFFECT OF TWO CONSECUTIVE SHIFTS OF AN $LD_{12:12}$ LIGHTI REGIMEN (A FIRST 6-HOUR [$-90° \Delta \phi s$] AND A SUBSEQUENT 12-HOUR PROLONGATION OF A SINGLE LIGHT SPAN [$-180° \Delta \phi s$]) ISOLATING STRAIN OR AGE DIFFERENCES IN SHIFT BEHAVIOR OF CIRCADIAN RHYTHM IN RECTAL TEMPERATURE OF INBRED CBA OR NZB MICE (ASSESSED BY CIRCADIAN ACROPHASE, ϕ*).

ANIMALS INVESTIGATED		COMPUTATIVE ACROPHASES ± 1.96 SE (ALL IN DEGREES)		
Mouse Strain	Age**	ϕ_1	ϕ_2	ϕ_3
NZB . CBA	Y	-349 ± 11	-74 ± 14	-217 ± 23
	O	-333 ± 19	-81 ± 28	-161 ± 25
NZB	Y	-342 ± 12	-70 ± 24	-192 ± 13
	O	-339 ± 16	-83 ± 20	-166 ± 21
CBA	Y	-331 ± 12	-71 ± 16	-136 ± 10
	O	-307 ± 19	-71 ± 31	-114 ± 24
A/JAX	Y	-346 ± 16	-58 ± 14	-149 ± 13
	O	-315 ± 22	-61 ± 25	-166 ± 20

*ϕ_1 = *Pre-shift acrophase ref. to 00^{00} local time ($L06^{00}$ - 18^{00}).*
ϕ_2 = *Day 4 post $-90° \Delta \phi s$ ($L06^{00}$ - 18^{00} to $L12^{00}$ - 00^{00} by prolongation of light) ϕ ref. is ϕ_1; target ϕ is 90° from ϕ_1.*
ϕ_3 = *Days 3 and 4 post $-180° \Delta \phi s$ ($L12^{00}$ - 00^{00} to $L00^{00}$ - 12^{00} by prolongation of light) ϕ ref. is ϕ_1; target ϕ is -270° from ϕ_1.*
**Y = *"Younger" animals (2-6 months of age); O = "older" animals (10-20 months of age).*

Whether one wants to give chlorothiazide in such a way as to enhance saluresis and diuresis and lower blood pressure while avoiding the detrimental kaliuresis and hypokalemia, or whether one wants to time the administration of an anti-cancer drug in such a fashion that the tumor can be hardest hit while the bone marrow is spared to the greatest extent possible, it will be extremely important to find a proper reference function to guide such critical timing. A most tempting, as yet unproved, candidate for this role of a "marker" function is body temperature. Major arguments for using temperature include the fact that it exhibits a rather reliable, i.e., stable, rhythm. Because of this stability, the timing of the temperature rhythm can serve as a ready reference for the timing of rhythms in other variables. Second, body core temperature can be monitored very easily with say, thermistors, thermocouples, or telemetry, the data being stored on small recorders. But even if it is self-measured with a clinical thermometer, circadian rhythms in temperature, if not ultradian ones, remain demonstrable in relatively sparse data. Finally, if even the single temperature measurement is deemed to be "too complex," one can simply record and time-code any laboratory determination or clinical observation by reference to the schedule of sleeping and working, on a rather simple form (Halberg, 1973). Thus, if a temperature record is unavailable, one should at least know, in dealing with a single blood sample withdrawn for clinical or research purposes, whether one deals with a night-shift worker or if the subject follows a diurnal activity, nocturnal rest schedule.

The plasma corticoid rhythms of several early risers as compared to those of the late risers are differently timed. Urinary corticoids may be a good marker for adrenal inhibition. In the case of breast cancers, changes in radiotracer uptake or variations in temperature over the hot spot of the breast should be monitored. For a tumor like a malignant plasmacytoma (multiple myeloma), Bence-Jones protein (found in the urine of about fifty percent of the patients) may, perhaps, constitute a reference function. Indeed, with Dr. Horace Zinneman (1974) we found cases with a circadian Bence-Jones protein excretion rhythm. If one plans chronotherapy on multiple myeloma one might, perhaps, have a ready reference function in urinary Bence-Jones protein rhythms. However, most urgently needed is a reference function for the human bone marrow. Peripheral (total and differential) blood cell counts and platelet counts and serum iron determinations are candidate markers, yet it remains uncertain whether any one or all of these will be sufficiently sensitive in one of their circadian rhythm stages to indicate a depletion of reserves. In any event, it is likely that many different kinds of rhythm-reference functions will be needed. The particular subsystem to be followed will determine the function to be investigated.

Dr. Reiter

I'm interested in the sensitivity of mice to ethanol. You reported that mice are more sensitive in the afternoon than they are in the morning to the same dose of ethanol when death rate is the endpoint. Is this a phenomenon that is influenced by photoperiod? The reason I'm asking this question is that we recently found that darkness is stimulatory to ethanol consumption in animals and that this is partially a function of the pineal gland (Reiter et al., 1973). I was wondering if there was a possibility that photoperiod is involved in the response you described. I'm also interested in your adrenal function study in the case of a hamster where the rhythm persisted for ten days. Were these cultured adrenals kept under constant conditions or was this perchance also influenced by the light-dark cycle? There is evidence that culture tissues can be directly influenced by photoperiod (Rosner et al., 1972).

Dr. Halberg

Ethanol effects in human beings have been studied by Rutenfranz and Singer (1967) and are currently being investigated by Dr. Erhard

Haus at Ramsey County Hospital, St. Paul. He found a remarkable rhythm in various aspects of ethanol metabolism and thus ethanol effect. Neither the recent studies of Haus nor similar studies carried out by Reinberg et al. (1974) in Paris bear directly upon the matter of ethanol preference.

Your point that animals are more sensitive to ethanol in the afternoon than in the morning is, of course, dependent on the lighting schedule. When death rate is determined on animals kept in light from 06^{00} to 18^{00}, a peak in ethanol susceptibility occurs around 20^{00} as demonstrated by Dr. Haus et al. (1959). If the lighting regimen is inverted, the peak is correspondingly displaced, as documented most recently by Nelson and Halberg (1973). Thus, the temporal placement of the daily photofraction is indeed a synchronizer of the murine susceptibility rhythm to ethanol.

However, if animals are placed in continuous darkness (Halberg, 1960), the ethanol rhythm persists with a circadian period slightly shorter than 24 hours. Accordingly, I suggested in 1960 that the rhythm can indeed be synchronized by light and darkness although it is not determined by this alternation as has been shown for many other rhythms. In any event, these rhythms in susceptibility to ethanol are so dramatic that they may serve as an excellent tool in your hands. You may wish to follow up our circadian studies on the ethanol susceptibility rhythm by a study of circannual changes in susceptibility to this agent. If such were readily demonstrated, one could then look at underlying circannual mechanisms which need not (but could) involve the pineal gland. By the same token, the possible involvement of the pineal gland in the dramatic circadian ethanol susceptibility rhythms indeed deserves study, as you suggest. I have no data in this connection.

I cannot answer your second question pertaining to the role of any periodicity of light and darkness in organ cultures. You prompt me to add that such periodicity may well have existed; the light exposure corresponded to the frequency of sampling times. Indeed it was frequent; it could have been a factor underlying a circadian rhythm by a frequency demultiplication of its effect. Thus, the circadian rhythm in organ cultures may well be synchronized by a sampling schedule with much higher frequency. I would be most interested in learning from you about any experience with (or reports on) direct effects of light that you know of with respect to organs in culture.

Dr. Craig

In some recent work, Dr. Harry Rounds (Witchita) has isolated a cardio-acceleratory factor that appears in the blood of cockroaches, rats, and man; and the interesting thing about it is it appears that it's regulated by the cycles of the moon or it shows up when the peak gravitation of the moon is in effect. Do you have any evidence or know of any evidence that correlates the pull of the moon with any circadian rhythms or any existing rhythms?

Dr. Halberg

In a number of human time series studies we find two components, one near 24.8 and another near 24.0 hours (Apfelbaum et al., 1969 and unpublished). If we turn to analyses by the inspection of records from human beings in isolation for several weeks, about 100 individuals studied by Aschoff et al. (1969), the average period is about 24.9 hours in length, again rather close to a lunar day. The original authors have emphatically noted that 24.9 in their data is statistically significantly different from 24.8 hours, yet the question that we confront is equally interesting whether we ask about the lunar component acquired in evolution and persisting as a second "free-running" component or whether this component can indeed be synchronized by some effect of the moon.

Professor William Luyten of the University of Minnesota and I have suggested (via channels) that an international cooperative study of the intraperitoneal temperature rhythm in a homeothermic mammal with a "lunar" period would be extremely interesting, not only at different distances from the moon but also on the moon itself.

Gravitationally, the moon causes tides on the earth -- in the oceans, in the atmosphere, and in the rocks. Since the moon has no oceans, and virtually no atmosphere, the only counterpart on the moon -- earth produced tides -- would be in the rocks.

The basic periodicity in lunar tides on earth is 24.8 hours; this is roughly the average time interval between meridian passages of the moon for any given place on earth. However, there is no similar periodicity in the gravitational effects of the earth on the moon since, for any given location on the moon, the earth would remain in nearly the same position in the sky relative to horizon and zenith, while the sun and the stars would appear to revolve behind it (in slightly different periods).

Moreover, for the sake of statistical and logistic (life support) considerations, it would be interesting to study orbital periods considerably shorter than those at 1/3 and 2/3 of the earth-moon distance. For example, if one used "Mercury" orbits (with a period of about 90 hours), one could look for an accentuated 90-hour rhythm. Orbital distances at which the periodicity of lunar exposure were say, non-harmonic with 24 hours (5,7,9...15) might give yet more decisive answers. If one went to the longer periods, one would have to be prepared to sustain the animals for a sufficient number of cycles to give a reliable period estimate.

Lunar effects on man and on other life forms have long been suspected in phenomena ranging from lunacy to agricultural practices. As yet, a direct causal relation has not been convincingly demonstrated for man and model mammals. The advent of orbital and lunar spaceflight now presents opportunities for a decisive investigation of this problem.

Under NASA sponsorship, as part of the former Biosatellite program, a system was developed for maintaining a group of rats in earth orbit for 3 weeks. During this time information on gross body movement, feeding activity, and body temperature was to be recorded on a nearly continuous basis and telemetered back to stations on earth. Techniques have also been developed for quantifying, testing, and displaying characteristics of rhythms in the data thus obtained. Using this system and these analytic methods, we proposed an investigation of circadian rhythms in rats exposed to lunar gravitational forces at different frequencies to determine whether or not the 24.8 hour periodicity exhibited by these animals on earth can be modified. Differences in periodicity of exposure to lunar influence would be achieved by differences in orbital characteristics. Furthermore, in what may be the most definitive step, this periodicity could be eliminated completely by stationing one of the animal packages on the moon itself.

It is in the latter feature of the proposed investigation that techniques developed by the USSR for soft-landing and retrieval of instrument packages would prove quite valuable.

With presumably minor modification, refurbishing, and updating, the former Biosatellite hardware, plus any additional units deemed scientifically desirable, could be put into service in orbital studies as part of the Skylab, the "orbiter" in the contracted Space Shuttle Program, or in some other form. On the other hand, extensive changes may be required to permit this hardware to function as a lunar station, yet the unique advantage of such a station in the investigation here discussed make the added effort and expense seem worthwhile.

DISCUSSION REFERENCES

Apfelbaum, M., Reinberg, A., Nillus, P., and Halberg, F. (1969). Presse Med. 77, 879-882.

Aschoff, J., Pöppel, E., and Wever, R. (1969). Pflügers Arch. 306, 58-70.

Bolles, R. and Duncan, P. (1969). Physiol. Behav. 4, 87.

Galicich, J. H., Halberg, F., and French, L. A. (1963). Nature 197, 811-813.

Galicich, J. H., Halberg, F., French, L. A., and Ungar, F. (1965). Endocrinol. 76, 895-901.

Halberg, E., Nelson, W., Scheving, L. E., Stupfel, M., Halberg, F., Bouquot, J. E., Vichers, R. A., and Gorlin, R. F. (1973). Int. J. Chronobiol. 1, 327-328.

Halberg, F. (1973). In: *Biological Aspects of Circadian Rhythms* (Mills, J. N., ed.), pp. 1-26, Plenum Press, New York.

Halberg, F. (1960). Cold Spring Harbor Symp. Quant. Biol. 25, 289-310.

Halberg, F., Galicich, J. H., Ungar, F., and French, L. A. (1965). Proc. Soc. Exp. Biol. Med. 118, 414-419.

Halberg, F., Halberg, E., Barnum, C. P., and Bittner, J. J. (1959). In: *Photoperiodism and Related Phenomena in Plants and Animals* (Withrow, R. B., ed.), pp. 803-878, Am. Assoc. Adv. Sci., Washington, D.C.

Halberg, F., Visscher, M. B., and Bittner, J. J. (1953). Am. J. Physiol. 174, 313-315.

Haus, E., Hanton, E. M., and Halberg, F. (1959). Physiologist 2, 54.

Levine, H., Halberg, F., and Taylor, D. (1973). Graefe's Archiv. 188, 263-280.

Levine, H., Ramshaw, W. A., and Halberg, F. (1967). Physiologist 10, 230 (Abstract).
Nelson, W., Cadotte, L., and Halberg, F. (1973). Proc. Soc. Exp. Biol. Med. 144, 766-769.
Nelson, W., Nichols, G., Halberg, F., and Kottke, G. (1973). Int. J. Chronobiol. 1, 347.
Nelson, W. and Halberg, F. (1973). Space Life Sci. 4, 249-257.
Pauly, J. E., Burns, E. R., Betterton, H., Tsai, S., Halberg, F., and Scheving, L. E. (1973). Int. J. Chronobiol. 1, 348-349.
Ramaley, J. A. (1974). Neuroendocrinology (In press).
Reinberg, A., Clench, J., Aymard, N., Galliot, M., Bourdon, R., Gervais, P., Abulker, C., and Dupont, J. (1974). C. R. Acad. Sci. Paris 278, 1503.
Reiter, R., Blum, K., Wallace, J., and Merritt, J. (1973). Quart. J. Stud. Alc. 34, 937-939.
Rosner, J., Denari, J., Nagle, C., Cardinali, D., de Perez Bedes, G., and Orsi, L. (1972). Life Sci. II (pt. II), 829-836.
Rutenfranz, J. and Singer, R. (1967). Int. Z. Angew. Physiol. Einschl. Arbeitsphysiol. 24, 1-17.
Stupfel, M., Halberg, E., and Halberg, F. (1973a). C. R. Acad. Sci. [D], Paris 277, 873-876.
Stupfel, M., Halberg, F., Halberg, F., Halberg, E., and Lee, J. K. (1973b). Int. J. Chronobiol. 1, 259-267.
Yunis, E. J., Halberg, F., McMullen, A., Roitman, B., and Fernandes, G. (1973). Int. J. Chronobiol. 1, 368-369.
Zinneman, H. H., Halberg, F., Haus, E., and Kaplan, M. (1974). Int. J. Chronobiol. 2, 3-16.

ENDOCRINE RHYTHMS ASSOCIATED WITH PINEAL GLAND FUNCTION

Russel J. Reiter

Department of Anatomy
Health Science Center
University of Texas at San Antonio
San Antonio, Texas 78284

OUTLINE

I. INTRODUCTION

The endocrine system exhibits a gamut of rhythms. Many of these have a duration of roughly 24 hours (circadian) while some are approxi-

---

Work by the author was supported in part by U.S.P.H.S. Grant HD-06523 and U.S.P.H.S. Career Development Award HD-42398.

mately 12 months (circannual) in length. All of the rhythms are probably advantageous to the individual animals or to the species as a whole. The factors controlling many of these hormonal fluctuations are likely numerous; and, in many cases, the governing mechanisms remain unknown. Some of the rhythms are undoubtedly related to the activity of the pineal gland, an organ which itself exhibits remarkable variations in its biosynthetic and presumably in its secretory activity. In the pineal gland, the primary impeller of these changes is ostensibly the photoperiodic environment (Quay, 1963a; Axelrod, Wurtman, and Snyder, 1965; Snyder, Axelrod, and Zweig, 1967) and to somewhat lesser extent locomotor activity (Ralph, Mull, Lynch, and Hedlund, 1971; Reiter, Sorrentino, Ralph, Lynch, Mull, and Jarrow, 1971) and hormonal feedback influences (Quay, 1964; Wurtman, Axelrod, Snyder, and Chu, 1965; Houssay and Barcello, 1972).

The present paper will consider those hormonal oscillations that may either directly or indirectly rely on the activity of the pineal gland. In some instances such relationships are well established while in others the evidence is tenuous or completely lacking. Before discussing these interactions, however, the nature of the pineal hormones and the evidence that the pineal gland exhibits regular fluctuations in activity will be summarized.

II. PINEAL HORMONES

1. Indoles

The pineal gland of all mammalian species examined is extremely rich in serotonin (5-hydroxytryptamine or 5-HT), and it also contains smaller quantities of related 5-hydroxy- and 5-methoxyindoles (Quay and Halevy, 1962; Quay, 1963b). The pineal constituent that has aroused the greatest interest among scientists is N-acetyl-5-methoxytryptamine (melatonin). Melatonin, an indole originally isolated from bovine pineal tissue (Lerner, Case, Takahashi, Lee, and Mori, 1958), is synthesized within the pineal gland by the N-acetylation of serotonin followed by the O-methylation of the product (Axelrod and Weissbach, 1960; Weissbach, Redfield, and Axelrod, 1960). The two enzymes required for these conversions are N-acetyltransferase and hydroxyindole-O-methyl transferase (HIOMT). Although the melatonin forming enzyme, HIOMT, was initially thought to be present only within the pineal gland, it has subsequently been identified within the mammalian retina (Cardinali and Rosner, 1971) and within the Harderian gland (Vlahakes and Wurtman, 1972; Cardinali and Wurtman, 1972). Despite the apparent lack of organ specificity of melatonin, it still commands attention as a pineal hormone.

In addition to converting serotonin to melatonin, the pineal can metabolize serotonin via other pathways as well. The primary route for the biotransformation of serotonin would appear to involve oxidative deamination in that relatively large amounts of 5-hydroxyindole acetic acid are found within pineal tissue (Quay, 1964). Likewise, the activity of monoamine oxidase, the enzyme that serves to deaminate serotonin, is characteristically high in mammalian pineals (Hakanson and Owman, 1966). The product of the deamination of serotonin is an unstable aldehyde intermediate, 5-hydroxyindole acetaldehyde, which may be oxidized to 5-hydroxyindole acetic acid or reduced to 5-hydroxytryptophol. These compounds can then be O-methylated by HIOMT to form 5-methoxyindole acetic acid and 5-methoxytryptophol, respectively (Axelrod and Weissbach, 1960). These latter two compounds have been isolated from pineal tissue (Lerner, Case, and Takahashi, 1960; McIsaac, Farrell, Taborsky, and Taylor, 1965) with 5-methoxytryptophol being present in rather high concentrations. The metabolic pathways of serotonin within the pineal gland are summarized in Figure 1.

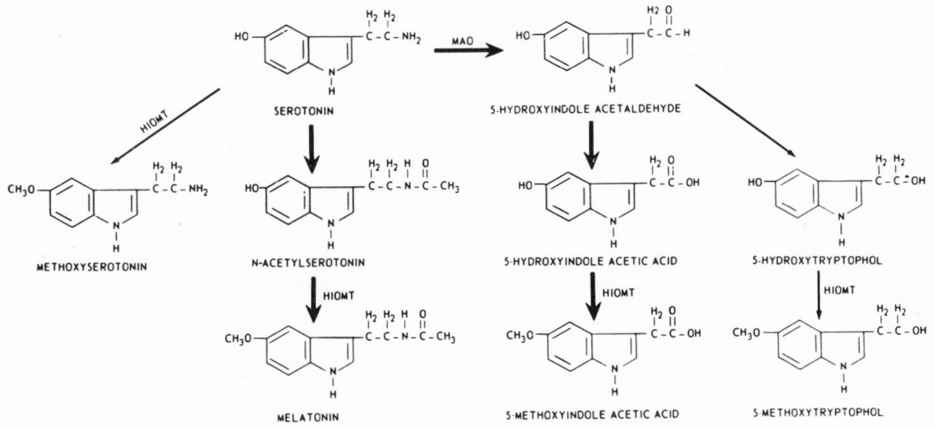

Figure 1. Metabolism of serotonin within the pineal gland. HIOMT: hydroxyindole-O-methyltransferase; MAO: monoamine oxidase.

A number of the pineal indoles have, at one time or another, been classified as pineal hormones. The indoles have been investigated primarily from the standpoint of their ability to inhibit gonadal development in immature rats or to depress reproductive functions in adult animals (Reiter, 1972a; 1973a). The first evidence which showed that melatonin acted as a hormone was provided by Wurtman, Axelrod, and Chu (1963). When injected daily into maturing female rats, it significantly retarded growth of the ovaries. Since then a raft of investigations have shown this indoleamine to possess gonad-inhibiting properties. When administered peripherally either by means of single (Vaughan, Benson, Norris, and Vaughan, 1971) or multiple (Moszkowska, 1965) injections or by subcutaneous implantation in beeswax (Rust and Meyer, 1969; Sorrentino, Reiter, and Schalch, 1971a), melatonin curtailed the growth of the gonads in both male and female mammals. It is also an effective inhibitor of ovulation (Longenecker and Gallo, 1971) and luteinizing hormone (LH) release (Reiter and Sorrentino, 1971) in immature rats induced to ovulate with pregnant mare's serum (PMS). Furthermore, when melatonin is applied directly to the neural structures which influence the anterior pituitary gland (Fraschini and Martini, 1970) or when it is infused into the cerebrospinal fluid (Kamberi, Mical, and Porter, 1971), it has a marked depressant effect on pituitary and plasma gonadotrophin levels. Although the majority of studies point to the antigonadotropic potential of melatonin, there are some workers who are not convinced that it is an active pineal hormone (Thieblot, Allassimare, and Blaise, 1966).

Melatonin is not the only pineal indole which has attained the status of a hormone. According to McIsaac, Taborsky, and Farrell (1964), 5-methoxytryptophol is somewhat more potent than melatonin in restricting gonadal maturation in rats when it is administered daily. When tested under other experimental conditions, 5-methoxytryptophol was found to specifically prevent the accumulation of follicle stimulating hormone (FSH) in the pituitary glands of castrated male rats (Fraschini and Martini, 1970) and to reduce by about one half compensatory growth of the ovary in unilaterally ovariectomized mice (Vaughan, Reiter, Vaughan, Bigelow, and Altschule, 1972). Albertazzi, Barbanti-Silva, Trentini, and Botticelli (1966) claimed that serotonin may be the factor which accounts for the antigonadotropic activity of the pineal gland; this suggestion is supported in part by the findings of Fraschini and Martini (1970). The precursor of melatonin, N-acetylserotonin, also restricts compensatory ovarian enlargement in mice (Vaughan et al., 1972); but, seemingly contradictory, it may release LH from the pituitary when it is infused into the cerebrospinal fluid (Porter, Mical, and Cramer, 1971/1972). Finally, 5-hydroxytryptophol has been shown to stymie the induced ovarian growth in mice which follows unilateral ovariectomy (Vaughan et al., 1972).

2. Polypeptides

Besides the indoles, polypeptides have captured considerable attention as being the dominant pineal secretory product. Generally less is known of their biochemical makeup and synthetic mechanisms, but physiologically their actions have been amply demonstrated. For at least two decades Thieblot and co-workers (Thieblot, 1965; Thieblot and Blaise, 1966; Thieblot and Menigot, 1971) have been trying to convince endocrinologists that the pineal is a polypeptide-secreting endocrine gland. The active fraction which they have isolated is believed to consist of five peptides and to have a molecular weight of 1,000-3,000 (Thieblot and Menigot, 1971). Its antigonadotropic potential seems unquestionable.

There are a number of other workers who are also enthusiastic about the peptidic nature of the pineal hormones. Moszkowska and Ebels (1971) and Ebels, Moszkowska, and Scemama (1970) extracted a number of constituents from bovine and ovine pineal powder. At least one of these fractions exhibited an inhibitory effect on pituitary FSH while another compound facilitated FSH release. The inhibitory polypeptide reportedly has a molecular weight somewhat less than that reported by Thieblot and Menigot (1971), being roughly in the range of 700.

The isolation of another polypeptide from acetone-dried powder of bovine pineal tissue was reported about 10 years ago by Milcu, Pavel, and Neascu (1963) and Pavel (1963). Because of its antidiuretic and oxytoxic activity, the compound was tentatively characterized as arginine vasotocin (AVT). In addition to these properties, the substance was found to be strongly inhibitory to gonadal growth in experimental animals. Further experimentation proved that the compound was in fact AVT (Cheesman, 1970; Pavel, 1971). Pavel, Petrescu, and Viocoleanu (1973) recently concluded that on the basis of the ability of AVT and melatonin to inhibit compensatory ovarian hypertrophy in mice the peptide is roughly a million times more potent than the indole (0.0001 μg AVT is equivalent to 100 μg melatonin). The potency of AVT in this test system has been confirmed by Vaughan and Klein (1973). There appears to be, however, some disagreement in terms of the level at which AVT acts, i.e., either centrally (Pavel *et al.*, 1973) or peripherally (Vaughan and Klein, 1973) or possibly both.

Several terms have been utilized to identify the active pineal polypeptide. Because of its ability to inhibit ovulation, Chazov and associates (Chazov, Isachenkov, Krisvosheyev, Veselova, and Zhivoderova, 1972) chose to call it anovulin. They theorized that they were dealing with an albumino-peptide. Benson, Matthews, and Rodin (1971, 1972) have elected to identify their pineal antigonadotropic material by the acronymic term PAG. Benson and colleagues have established that their PAG is melatonin-free and is probably a polypeptide. It is considered to be 60-70 times more potent than melatonin in inhibiting compensatory enlargement of the ovary in unilaterally ovariectomized mice, and it is believed to have a molecular weight between 500-1000. They have concluded that the PAG is not identical with the pineal arginine vasotocin which has been isolated by other workers (Cheesman, 1970; Pavel, 1971). The physiological effects of PAG have recently been reviewed (Benson and Orts, 1972).

The issue of the biochemical nature of the active pineal antigonadotropic principle(s) requires resolution before researchers can define the complex physiological effects of the pineal gland. It is possible, however, that both indoles and polypeptides are secreted by this ubiquitous-acting endocrine gland. Certainly the two groups are not mutually exclusive.

III. PINEAL RHYTHMS

The mammalian pineal is richly endowed with serotonin and norepinephrine (NE). The organ also contains large amounts of the enzymes required for the synthesis and metabolism of these important biogenic amines. Within the pineal gland many of the constituents undergo daily fluctuations. One important factor determining these oscillations is the prevailing environmental photoperiod acting by way of the sympathetic nervous system.

1. Daily Rhythms

a. Norepinephrine

The concentration of NE in the pineal gland of the rat ranges from 3-12 μg/g (Wurtman, Axelrod, Sedvall, and Moore, 1967). The catecholamine is almost exclusively confined to the postganglionic nerve terminals which abound in the pineal gland (Zieher and Pellegrino de Iraldi, 1966). Pineal NE exhibits a pronounced diurnal rhythm, being about 3 times higher during darkness than during light (Wurtman and Axelrod, 1966) (Figure 2).

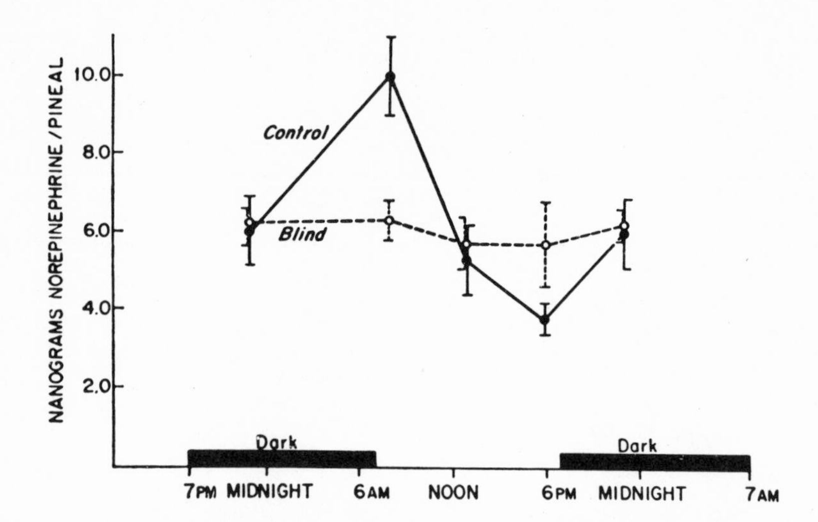

Figure 2. Daily rhythm in norepinephrine in the pineal gland of intact and blinded rats. Data from Wurtman and Axelrod (1966).

The rhythm in pineal NE is abolished by depriving animals of light or by placing them under continuous illumination. Thus, the rhythm seems to be exogenous and is generated by environmental light. The rate limiting enzyme in the synthesis of NE, tyrosine hydroxylase, also fluctuates in a circadian manner and is higher at night than during the day (McGeer and McGeer, 1966). The other enzymes required for the synthesis of NE from tyrosine have also been found in the pineal along with monoamine oxidase and catechol-O-methyltransferase, the two enzymes which serve to catabolize NE.

When pineal NE is released, it causes a dramatic effect within the pinealocytes. Catecholamines generally appear to produce their actions by stimulating the synthesis of 3'5'-cyclic adenosine monophosphate. This compound has received considerable attention as an intracellular mediator of hormonal actions. Adenyl cyclase activity is relatively high in the pineal gland (Weiss and Costa, 1967); and since it is not influenced by superior cervical ganglionectomy, it is considered to be located postsynaptically. Norepinephrine stimulates pineal adenyl cyclase while exposure of experimental animals to continuous light reduces the activity of the enzyme. The findings suggest that during light exposure NE is probably not released from the pineal sympathetic nerves.

b. Serotonin

The concentration of serotonin in the pineal gland is several times higher than in any other mammalian organ (Giarman, Freedman, and Picardi-Ami, 1960; Quay and Halevy, 1962). Although at birth the levels are very low, the adult levels of the amine are attained during the second week of life. Like NE, serotonin exhibits a circadian variation within the pineal gland (Quay, 1963a; Illnerova, 1971) (Figure 3). However, the

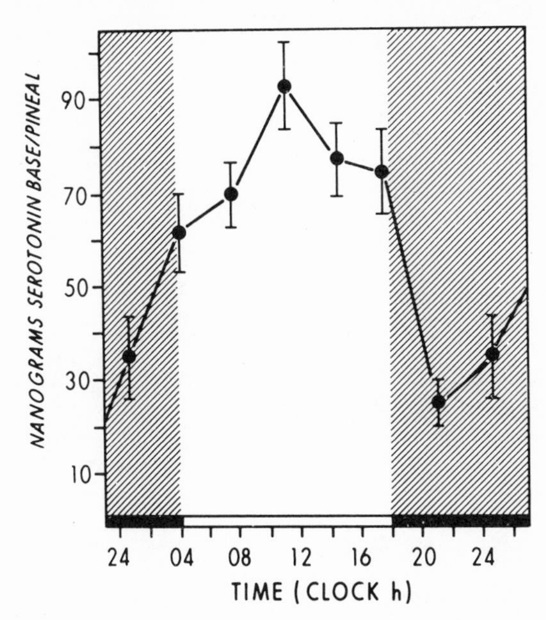

Figure 3. Diurnal variation in serotonin within the pineal gland of adult male rats. Cross-hatched areas indicate period of darkness. Data from Quay (1963a).

serotonin rhythm is inversely related to that for NE, being elevated during the light phase and depressed during the dark phase. The serotonin rhythm persists during light deprivation but is abolished by constant light exposure (Quay, 1963a). Sympathetic denervation of the pineal gland extinguishes the serotonin rhythm.

Neither the rates of hydroxylation of tryptophan nor the decarboxylation of 5-hydroxytryptophan nor the activity of monoamine oxidase seem to have much to do with the circadian cycle of serotonin (Snyder, Axelrod, and Zweig, 1967). On the other hand, the activity of _N_-acetyltransferase, the enzyme which converts serotonin to _N_-acetylserotonin, may play a significant role in this regard.

The conversion of serotonin to _N_-acetylserotonin via the action of _N_-acetyltransferase is extremely active in pineals of animals killed during darkness. In fact, Klein and associates (Klein and Weller, 1970; Klein, Reiter, and Weller, 1971) have shown that, compared to daytime values, the activity of the acetylating enzyme increases 15-60 fold at night (Figure 4). This rhythm is 180° out of phase with that of sero-

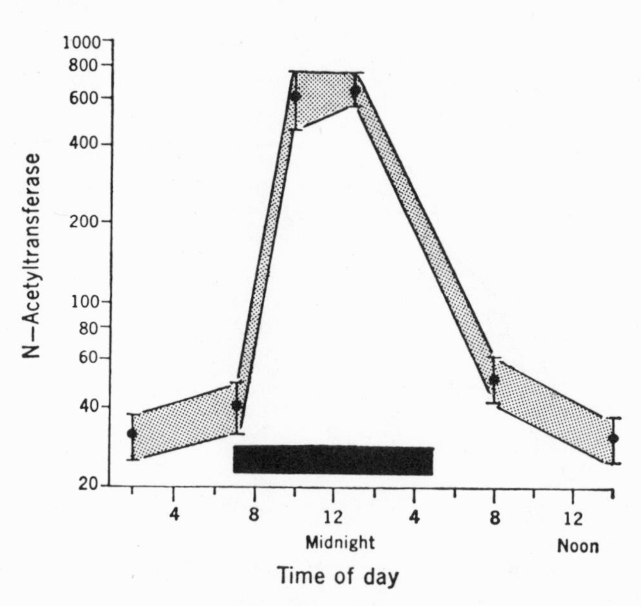

Figure 4. Daily rhythm in N-acetyltransferase within the rat pineal gland. The black bar represents the period of darkness. Enzyme activity is given as the number of picomoles of [^{14}C] serotonin N-acetylated per gland homogenate per hour. Data from Klein and Weller (1970).

tonin and corresponds closely with that of NE and melatonin. Klein and Weller (1970) argue convincingly that the activity of N-acetyltransferase is rate limiting in melatonin formation.

c. Melatonin

As already mentioned, the product of the acetylation of serotonin, N-acetylserotonin, is methylated by hydroxyindole-O-methyltransferase (HIOMT) to form melatonin (Axelrod and Weissbach, 1960). Under photic conditions of 12 hours of light alternating with 12 hours of darkness, pineal HIOMT activity is highest during the dark phase (Wurtman, Axelrod, and Phillips, 1963; Axelrod, Wurtman, and Snyder, 1965) (Figure 5). This rhythm is abolished by constant light exposure; but, contrary to some reports (Axelrod *et al.*, 1965), it probably persists during prolonged darkness. Likewise, removal of the superior cervical ganglia obliterates the rhythm in HIOMT (Wurtman, Axelrod, and Fischer, 1964).

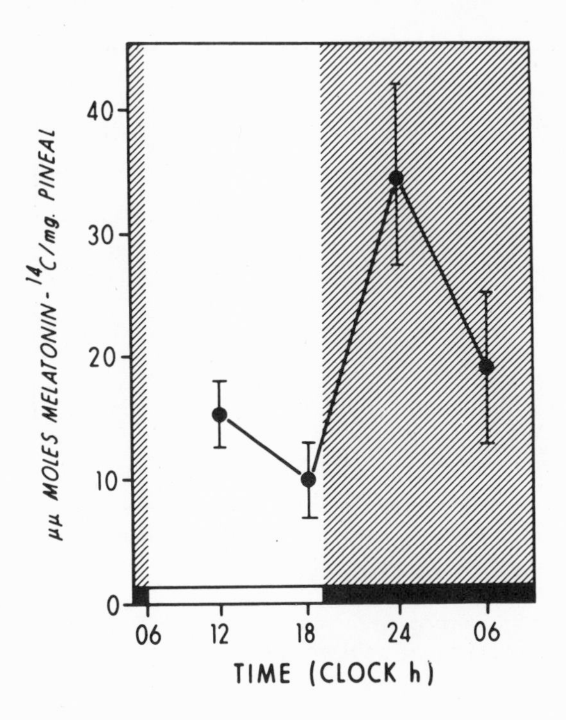

Figure 5. Diurnal variation in hydroxyindole-O-methyltransferase activity in the pineal gland of adult rats. Cross-hatched areas indicate period of darkness. Data from Axelrod et al. (1965).

The concentration of melatonin itself within the pineal gland follows very closely the activity of both N-acetyltransferase and HIOMT. Predictably, when the conversion of serotonin to melatonin is activated by darkness, melatonin accumulates within the pineal gland. Quay (1964) was the first to describe the circadian rhythm of melatonin in the rat pineal. Subsequent studies have shown that a similar diurnal fluctuation in pineal melatonin exists in the hamster (Reiter, 1974a), in the Japanese quail (Coturnix coturnix japonica) and in the White Leghorn chicken (Gallus domesticus) (Lynch, 1971). Figure 6 summarizes melatonin rhythms in the pineal of the rat and the two avian species. One of the most interesting features of the cyclic changes in pineal melatonin content is that the oscillations persist in blinded or continuously dark-exposed rats; and under these conditions, the rhythms are phase-locked with the free-running, circadian rhythms of locomotor activity (Ralph, Mull, Lynch, and Hedlund, 1971; Reiter, Sorrentino, Ralph, Lynch, Mull, and Jarrow, 1971). Furthermore, the amplitude of the rhythm in blinded rats is similar to that of rats kept in alternating light-dark cycles.

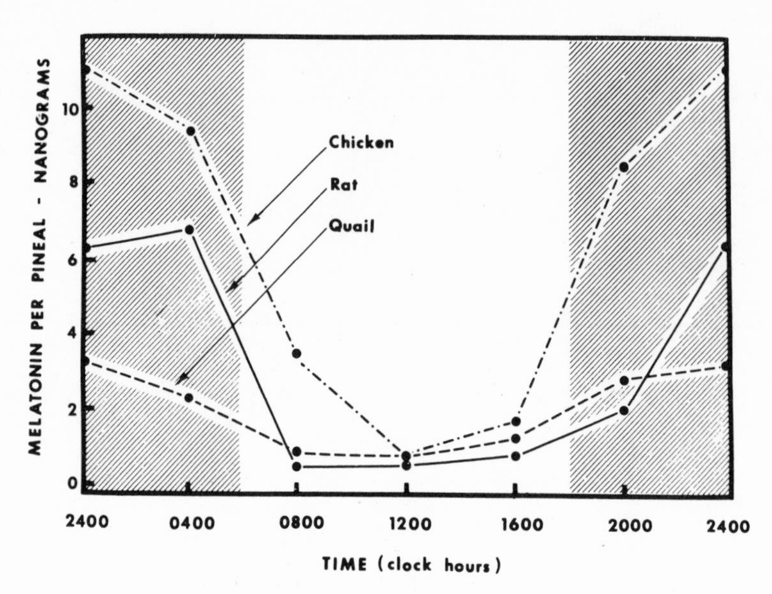

Figure 6. Daily variation in the melatonin content of pineals of three species of vertebrates. Cross-hatched areas indicate period of darkness. Data from Lynch (1971).

High locomotor activity in the light-deprived animal is correlated with elevated pineal melatonin content.

If melatonin accounts exclusively for the gonad-inhibiting activity of the pineal gland, then it could logically be assumed that pineals of animals killed during darkness would possess more antigonadotropic potential than pineals from animals killed during the light phase of the light-dark cycle. M. K. Vaughan, however, found this not to be the case. Indeed, single pineal glands from dark-killed and light-killed rats inhibit compensatory ovarian hypertrophy in mice with equal facility; and in each case a dose response curve was established. These observations were discussed in a recent review (Reiter, Vaughan, Vaughan, Sorrentino, and Donofrio, 1974).

This finding raises several interesting questions. The results seem to indicate that the pineal gland of the blinded animal produces no more melatonin than that of a rat kept in alternating light-dark cycles. Why, then is the pineal of the light-deprived rat more strongly antigonadotropic (Reiter, 1968a)? Does this mean that melatonin is not the pineal factor which forces gonadal regression in blinded animals? Possibly some other gonad-inhibiting factor is produced in much greater amounts during prolonged darkness. Unfortunately, since we know very little about the secretory rate of melatonin, or for that matter any of the other pineal constituents, these questions cannot be presently answered.

We do, however, know that melatonin gets into the systemic circulation. The indoleamine has been identified in the blood of the chicken (Pelham, Ralph, and Campbell, 1972) where it exhibits a diurnal variation, highest during darkness (Pelham and Ralph, 1972). Following pinealectomy melatonin is no longer detectable in the peripheral circulation. Presumptive melatonin has also been identified in the blood of normal adult male humans (aged 20-32 years) (Pelham, Vaughan, Sandock, and Vaughan, 1973). For this study human volunteers were housed under rigidly controlled light-dark conditions (14 hours of light and 10 hours of darkness daily). Analyses of repeated blood samples revealed that melatonin was not present in detectable amounts during the light hours but was easily detectable at night (Figure 7). Hence, the melatonin cycle in the

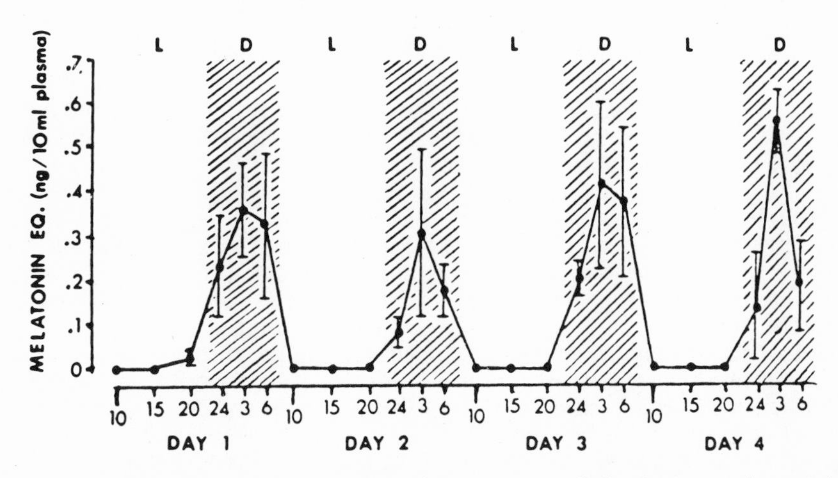

Figure 7. Melatonin rhythm in the plasma of 5 adult human male subjects. Activity within plasma is expressed as melatonin equivalents in mg/10 ml plasma. Cross-hatched areas represent periods of darkness. Data from Pelham et al. (1973).

human seems to be very similar to that in experimental animals.

Virtually nothing is known of the synthesis of the polypeptides within the pineal. Whether the elaboration of these compounds is dark-dependent or exhibits any functionally significant rhythms remains to be established.

Using indole synthesis within the pineal gland as an index of general activity, it is obvious that the metabolic rate fluctuates with the phase of the light-dark cycle. Specifically, the data imply greater activity during darkness. Presuming that all the pineal principles are secreted during the period of active synthesis, the pineal would exert its primary effects on the endocrine system either during the night or during prolonged periods of short photoperiods, such as during the winter months. This generally appears to be the case as will be discussed in the subsequent sections of this report.

2. Rhythms Associated with the Estrous Cycle

The information in this area is relatively sparse. In addition to the well-documented circadian variation in pineal serotonin, Quay (1963a) also reported that pineal serotonin content was lowest (statistically insignificant) at midday of proestrus in the rat. The estrous rhythm of 5-hydroxyindole acetic acid is opposite to that of serotonin, being lowest on the last day of diestrus and highest during proestrus and estrus (Quay, 1964). According to Wurtman, Axelrod, Snyder, and Chu (1965), the activity of the melatonin forming enzyme, HIOMT, is greatest on the days of diestrus and drops to half this value during proestrus and estrus. The implication is that ovarian steroids may feed back on the pineal and determine the ability of the organ to produce melatonin. Unfortunately, the melatonin rhythm does not correlate with the estrous variation of serotonin. If melatonin synthesis is lowest during proestrus or estrus, one would expect serotonin to be elevated rather than depressed. When specifically investigated, estradiol was able to inhibit NE-induced adenyl cyclase activity in the pineal, suggesting a site of feedback action of ovarian steroids (Weiss and Crayton, 1970).

3. Annual Rhythms

Primarily only morphological data are available to support the concept of change in pineal function with the season of the year. However, on the basis of what we know about photoperiodic length and pineal biosynthetic processes, it seems safe to predict that animals which are exposed to natural photoperiods would possess more highly functional pineal glands during the winter (short day) months. This would be especially true of animals (or humans) which live at the extremes of latitude where seasonal daylength varies most markedly. It is also important to consider pineals of fossorial species which are also nocturnal in nature. Certainly, such animals are exposed to only short photoperiods each day, regardless of the season. Finally, hibernatory species may not witness any light whatsoever for months during their hibernatory phase. Presuming the pineals of these animals are functional, these organs must become physiologically important under these conditions. In view of this, more studies on pineal biochemistry as a function of season should be conducted.

Almost two decades ago, Quay (1956) carried out careful histophysiological studies on the pineal gland of the white-footed mouse (Peromyscus leucopus) and concluded that the pineal is probably related to the antigonadotropic capability of short photoperiods. About the same time Pflügfelder (1956) and Mogler (1958) were examining seasonal variations in the endocrine glands, including the pineal, of hamsters which had been maintained under a natural photoperiodic environment. After meticulously measuring nuclear sizes of the pinealocytes and correlating these observations with the functional status of the testes, they theorized that the pineal was functionally most active during the short day (winter) months and that the activity of the pineal was inversely related to the status of the gonads, i.e., high pineal activity was accompanied by involution of the testes and vice versa. In another species, the ewe, histochemical studies also revealed that the gland was most active in December, January, and February (Nesić, 1962).

Animals that normally inhabit either the arctic or antarctic regions have unique pineal glands in many respects. Most importantly, they are extremely large compared to pineals of related species which reside in the temperate or tropical zones. For example, the Weddell seal (Leptonichotes weddelli), an aquatic carnivor, has a pineal gland roughly five times larger than that in a human (Figure 8) and about eight times

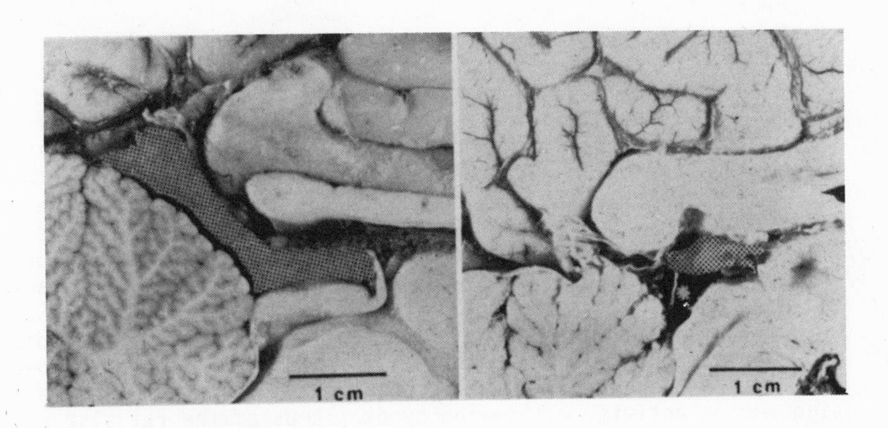

Figure 8. Pineal glands (stippled areas) from a Weddell seal (left) and from a human (right). Photos are the same magnification. The superior cisterna (*) is seen in the human brain. From Cuello and Tramezzani (1969).

larger than those of similarly sized carnivors which are restricted to temperate zones (Cuello and Tramezzani, 1969). Struck with the interesting features of this enormous gland, Cuello and Tramezzani (1969) concluded that the seasonal histochemical changes in the pineal of the Weddell seal must surely be related to the annual sexual cycle of the animal. These size relationships also hold true for the walrus (Turner, 1888), penguin (Watzka and Voss, 1967), and the northern fur seal (Elden, Keyes, and Marshall, 1971). Like Cuello and Tramezzani (1969), Elden et al. (1971) feel strongly that the remarkable pineal in the northern fur seal is related to its pelagic and seasonally reproductive nature. Conception in this species characteristically occurs during the month of July when long days prevail (minimal pineal activity?). When HIOMT levels were measured in the pineals of the seal, they had the capability to form 3 to 5 times more melatonin than pineals of humans. However, this may again be placing unwarranted emphasis on the importance of melatonin, since the nature of the antigonadotropic factor in this, or for that matter any other, species still remains unknown.

IV. EXTRA-PINEAL ENDOCRINE RHYTHMS

Rhythmic fluctuations of animals in their natural habitat are obvious features to experimental endocrinologists. The internal physiological "clock" which underlies these rhythms is, in many cases, far from clarified. Rhythms in which external environmental stimuli, especially photoperiod, participate may well involve the pineal gland as an intermediate or it may serve as a driving force for the rhythm.

1. Daily Rhythms

a. Adrenal

Probably one of the most thoroughly investigated of all endocrine rhythms has been that of corticosterone secretion by the adrenal cortex. In rats maintained in 12 to 14 hours of light per day, non-stressed plasma corticosterone levels are usually 2-6 times higher in the afternoon than in the morning (Dunn, Dyer, and Bennett, 1972). This 24-hour rhythm seems to develop in rats about 3 to 4 weeks of age (Allen and Kendall, 1967; Ramaley, 1973), which corresponds roughly to the age at which the pineal rhythms appear. Constant light exposure, which is inhibitory to pineal function, reportedly obliterates the afternoon peak in plasma corticosterone and suppresses the rhythmic secretion of adrenocorticotropin from the pituitary (Cheifez, Gaffud, and Dingman, 1968). However, in that constant light has direct effects on the neuroendocrine axis, the above results do not necessarily establish a connection between the pineal gland and adrenal rhythmic phenomena. Adrenocorticotropin releasing factor activity within the hypothalamus of the rat also exhibits a circadian periodicity (Hiroshige, Abe, Wada, and Kaneko, 1973). This fluctuation persists after bilateral removal of the superior cervical ganglia, a procedure which is believed to render the pineal gland non-functional (Reiter, 1972b).

When light deprivation was used in an attempt to alter adrenal function the results were variable. According to Jacobs and Kendall (1972), blinding suppressed the afternoon rise in plasma corticosterone unless the rats were pinealectomized. On the other hand, Dunn, Bennett, and Peppler (1972) found that morning and afternoon non-stressed levels of corticosterone in rats were not influenced by blinding and anosmia. Usually dual sensory deprivation (blindness plus anosmic) is considered to be maximally stimulatory to the pineal gland (Reiter, 1973a). It appears that if the pineal gland does participate in determining the cyclic functioning of the hypothalamo-pituitary-adrenal axis, proof of this will have to await further experimentation.

b. Growth hormone

A circadian pattern for pituitary and plasma growth hormone (GH) in rats was reported by Muller, Guistina, Miedico, Pecile, Cocchi, and King (1970). When GH was measured by both bioassay and radioimmunoassay, the results clearly showed that pituitary levels of growth hormone gradually increased throughout the day to a peak at 1800-2100 hours (Figure 9). The onset of darkness initiated a sustained drop in pituitary GH levels. Plasma growth hormone titers exhibited wide fluctuations with the peak concentrations being reached at 1800 and again at 0300 hours. Despite

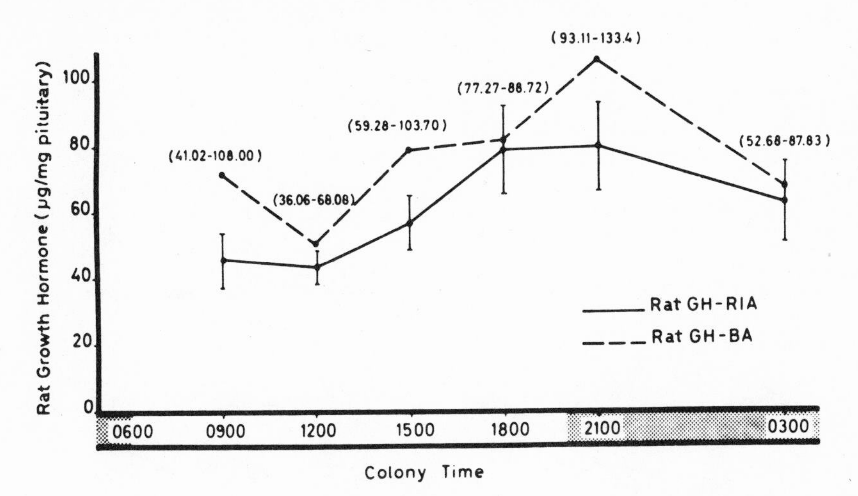

Figure 9. Diurnal rhythm of bioassayable (BA) and radioimmunoassayable (RIA) growth hormone (GH) in female rats. Shaded area indicates period of darkness. Numbers in parentheses represent 95% fiducial limits for BA-GH. Data from Muller et al. (1970).

the fact that pineal-GH interactions have been extensively studied (Sorrentino, Schalch, and Reiter, 1971b), the relationships between the circadian variation in GH and, e.g., pinealectomy, have never been investigated.

c. Prolactin

Pituitary and plasma prolactin levels undergo daily cyclic variations. Clark and Baker (1964) observed that bioassayable (pigeon crop assay) pituitary prolactin content in rats was highest during the light phase of the light-dark cycle. Meanwhile, plasma prolactin titers are inversely related to the pituitary rhythm with blood levels being highest during darkness. This has been noticed in the male rat (Rønnekleiv, Krulich, and McCann, 1973), in the pregnant (Butcher, Fugo, and Collins, 1972) and pseudopregnant rat (Freeman and Neill, 1972), and also in humans (Sassin, Frantz, Weitzman, and Kapen, 1972). The diurnal rhythm in plasma prolactin titers was extinguished in pinealectomized rats, suggesting darkness modifies prolactin secretion by an action on the pineal gland (Rønnekleiv et al., 1973) (Figure 10). Indeed, the pineal gland in light-deprived rats has been shown to strongly depress pituitary prolactin levels, probably by preventing the production or release of prolactin inhibiting factor (Donofrio and Reiter, 1972). The effects of the pineal on prolactin may be mediated by melatonin (Kamberi, Mical, and Porter, 1971).

d. Gonadotropins

Variations in the daily secretory activity of gonadotropins have been extensively reported in the last 15 years (Everett, 1961; Martini,

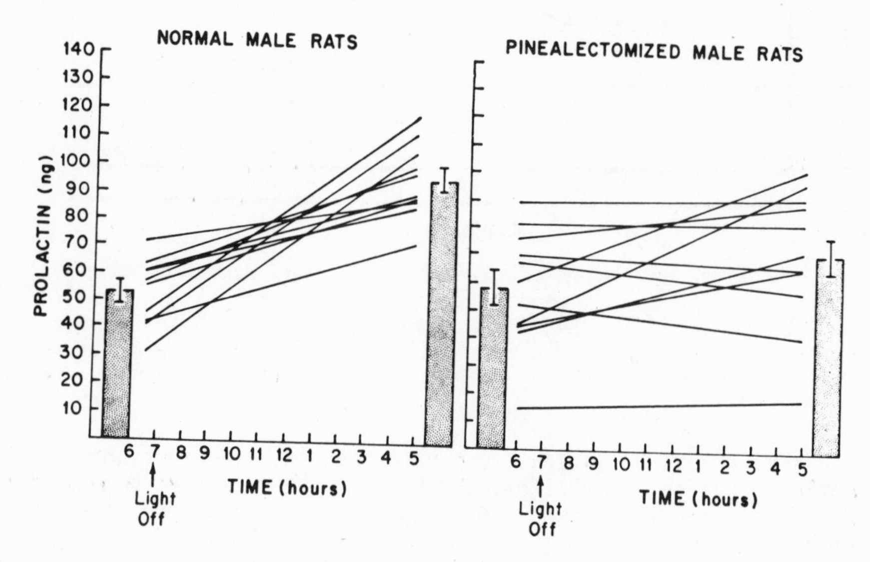

Figure 10. Variations in serum prolactin levels in intact male rats bled at 6 p.m. and 5 a.m. (left) compared to prolactin levels in pinealectomized rats bled at the same time (right). Data from Rønnekleiv et al. (1973).

Fraschini, and Motta, 1968; Schwartz, 1970). In male rats the cycle has a diurnal periodicity whereas in females, although it may exist, it is partially masked by the cyclic changes associated with ovulation. In male Sprague-Dawley rats, the peaks for pituitary FSH and LH were found to occur in the afternoon (Fraschini and Martini, 1970). Plasma levels of LH also exhibited diurnal fluctuations with titers being highest during the light phase of the light-dark cycle (Lawton and Schwartz, 1968; Dunn, Arimura, and Scheving, 1972).

According to F. Fraschini (unpublished observations) superior cervical ganglionectomy abolishes the decrease in pituitary LH and FSH concentration which usually occurs near the middle of the dark period. Since ganglionectomy functionally denervates the pineal gland, this finding could be interpreted as being a result of a lack of pineal function in these animals. Hypothalamic deafferentation also negates the rhythm in pituitary LH and FSH (Simonovic, Tima, and Martini, 1971). The authors suggest, as one of the explanations for their results, that the pineal can no longer influence the pituitary after the hypothalamus is disconnected from the remainder of the brain since the pineal normally modifies the pituitary secretion of gonadotropins by means of an extra-hypothalamic locus. Although deafferentation is capable of negating any effect of the pineal on the pituitary (Reiter, 1972b), the findings of Simonovic _et al_. (1971) have other explanations which are equally as tenable.

2. Rhythms Associated with the Estrous Cycle

The changes in LH and FSH as a function of the sexual cycle have already been alluded to. The pineal indole, melatonin, is capable of inhibiting spontaneous or induced ovulation and LH release in rats (Reiter and Sorrentino, 1971; Ying and Greep, 1973), suggesting that the pineal gland has the capability of modifying the estrous cycle. Rats that are rendered blind and anosmic and hamsters that are blinded only either exhibit extremely erratic estrous cycles or are completely acyclic (Reiter, Sorrentino, and Ellison, 1970; Sorrentino and Reiter, 1970). These effects of light deprivation or light deprivation and anosmia are overcome by pinealectomy.

Rats exposed to alternating cycles of 14 hours of light and 10 hours of darkness release an ovulatory surge of LH and ovulate every 4 or 5 days (Schwartz and McCormack, 1972). Both of these events, i.e., the LH release and ovulation are carefully regulated, occur at a specific time during the light-dark cycle and are photoperiodically controlled. Because of the close connection of spontaneous ovulation and photoperiod, it was a natural setting in which to test the influence of the pineal gland. When examined, pinealectomy was found to have no effect on the timing of the ovulatory mechanisms in adult female rats (Alleva, Waleski, and Alleva, 1970). A similar lack of an effect of pineal removal on ovulation has been obtained in hamsters although in this species continuous light exposure did alter the timing of the LH surge (Morin, 1973). This shows, as previously mentioned, that not all of the effects of constant light on the neuroendocrine axis are due to an inhibition of pineal function; there are certainly direct effects as well.

3. Annual Rhythms

One of the physiological niches which the pineal seems to have is to synchronize the reproductive periods of seasonal breeding species (at least in those in which this has been tested) to the proper season of the year. Correlating birth of the young with the spring or early summer is essential since it ensures maximal chances of survival of the young and, thereby, permits perpetuation of the species (Reiter, 1973a). Since it is a function of the pineal gland to correlate breeding activity with seasonal photoperiodic changes, the pineal obviously becomes indispensible for survival, not so much for survival of the individual animal but rather for survival of the species.

About 10 years ago the functional relationships between the prevailing environmental photoperiod and pineal activity were demonstrated (Quay, 1963a; Wurtman, Axelrod, and Phillips, 1963). Generally, the absence of light seems to exaggerate at least certain aspects of pineal function. In a highly photosensitive species, the golden hamster (Mesocricetus auratus), this interaction can be readily illustrated. When hamsters are subjected to total or near total light deprivation, the neuroendocrine-gonadal axis collapses and reproductive involution ensues (Hoffman and Reiter, 1965). Probably the most remarkable aspect of the change in the functioning of the hypothalamo-pituitary-gonadal axis is that the reproductive atrophy is totally prevented by removal of the pineal gland, which in the hamster weighs approximately 0.5 mg. This initial study was followed by a series of investigations which were designed to elucidate the function of the pineal gland under experimental and more physiological conditions.

Unless pinealectomized or superior cervical ganglionectomized (a procedure which renders the pineal non-functional), the blinding of adult male or female hamsters leads to regression of their gonads and adnexa to an infantile state within 6-8 weeks. After the regression is completed, for at least a short time thereafter, both the pineal gland and its functional innervation must be left intact to "hold" the gonads in a regressed condition (Reiter, 1968b). With long term light deprivation, however, the influence of the pineal gland on the neuroendocrine axis becomes readjusted. After approximately 20-25 weeks, the pineal can no longer maintain the sexual organs in the regressed state, and as a result, they spontaneously regenerate (Hoffman, Hester, and Towns, 1965; Reiter, 1968b).

This phenomenon of spontaneous regeneration was initially unexpected. However, examination of the data revealed that the period of reproductive collapse corresponded roughly in length to the winter interval of sexual dormancy of this species under field conditions. Golden hamsters are hibernators and seasonal breeders. Under natural conditions they enter hibernation in the fall of the year with regressed gonads and emerge from hibernation the following spring (Smit-Vis, 1972). Of course, during the hibernatory period the animals are normally underground in completely lightless burrows. An interesting feature of the seasonal sexual cycle is that near the end of hibernation (as spring approaches), the gonads begin to regenerate even though the hamsters are confined to total darkness (Smit-Vis and Akkerman-Bellaart, 1967). Thus, when the animals emerge from their burrows in the spring, they are immediately capable of reproducing. This natural cycle is very similar to that described in the light-deprived hamsters kept under laboratory conditions (Reiter, 1968b). In this situation, darkness induces gonadal regression which is followed eventually by spontaneous gonadal regeneration. Hence, the cycle observed under experimental conditions seems to simulate the normal reproductive cycle of the animal.

This presumed relationship led us to test the relationship between the pineal gland and the photoperiodically-regulated annual reproductive cycle more thoroughly. After the spontaneous restoration of the genital apparatus, the system does not experience a second decline in function as long as the animals are maintained in the absence of photic stimuli (Reiter, 1969). Conversely, if hamsters are deprived of light for a 30-week period (during which time the gonads regress and spontaneously regenerate) and are then exposed to long photoperiods (14 hours light per day, simulated summer), their return to darkness is followed by regression of the sexual organs (Reiter, 1972c). For this to occur, however, the simulated summer must be about 22 weeks in length (Figure 11). In

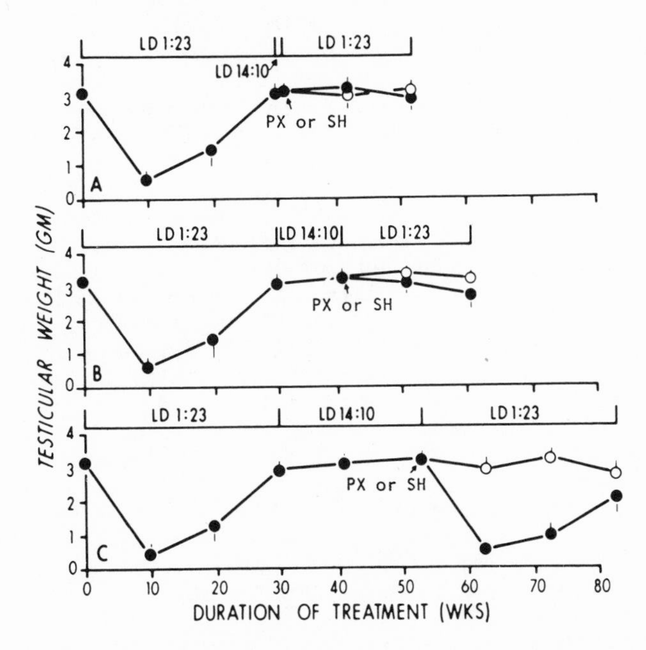

Figure 11. Effect of exposure of hamsters to L14:D10 cycles after an initial 30-week period of exposure to L1:D23 for either one (A), ten (B) or 22 (C) weeks on the subsequent degenerative response of the testes to short photoperiods. Solid points indicate intact or sham (SH) operated hamsters and hollow points indicate testicular sizes in pinealectomized (PX) hamsters. Data from Reiter (1972c).

this experimental situation we presumably duplicated what happens normally to this species under field conditions. The initial exposure to darkness (representing the fall of the year when the animals enter lightless burrows in preparation for hibernation) was followed by regression of the reproductive organs. After 25 weeks the gonads regenerated (representing the spring regeneration in preparation for the breeding season); and when they were exposed to L14:D10 (representing their emergence from hibernation), the hamsters already had functionally mature gonads. During the simulated summer months the gonads were refractory to inhibition by darkness acting via the pineal gland. However, if the simulated summer was extended for 22 weeks (1 year from the onset of the experiment), the pineal again became capable of inducing reproductive atrophy. This suggests that hamsters normally breed, or are at least capable of doing so, throughout the summer. The 22 weeks of photoperiodic stimulation during the summer seems to play a key role in "breaking" the period of summer refractoriness.

When subjected to test, the relationships described for hamsters under experimental conditions were similar to those in hamsters kept under natural photoperiodic and temperature conditions. If, in November, adult male hamsters were placed in a natural environment, their reproductive organs were completely regressed in January (Reiter, 1973b). By comparison, pinealectomized controls killed at the same time had grossly and histologically normal testes (Figure 12). By mid-March the gonads of the intact hamsters exhibited considerable regeneration whereas those of the pinealectomized hamsters were still normal in appearance. Regeneration of the gonads in the intact hamsters was completed soon thereafter; and, as predicted, during the subsequent summer months, exposure of the hamsters to darkness did not initiate gonadal atrophy, i.e., the system was refractory to the inhibitory influence of the pineal gland.

We have subsequently found that pinealectomized hamsters in natural photoperiodic environments, in addition to maintaining their reproductive organs in a functionally mature condition during the winter months, also are capable of successful breeding (Reiter, 1974b). When pinealectomized females were caged with pinealectomized males beginning in late December, the females became pregnant and delivered young during January and February. Intact hamsters, however, were not capable of reproducing until March (Figure 13), the time at which their gonads regenerated. Thus, the pineal is indeed capable of determining when hamsters, which are exposed to natural photoperiods, are able to deliver their young. Ensuring that the pups are born in the spring has obvious survival implications. The relationships between the photoperiod, the pineal, and annual reproductive performance in the golden hamster have recently been reviewed (Reiter, 1973a).

The golden hamster is not the only species in which the pineal gland seems to be inextricably linked with annual reproductive changes. In the Djungarian hamster (*Phodopus sungorus* Pallas) as well, a winter decline in the size of the gonads is apparent (Hoffmann, 1972; 1973). This species also exhibits a seasonal change in body weight and pelage color, being gray to black in the summer and nearly white in the winter. All these changes are related to the photoperiod with short daily light

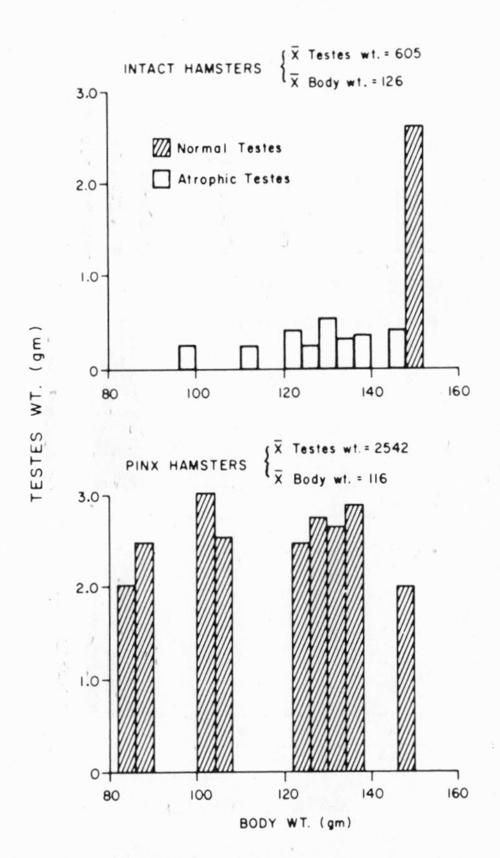

Figure 12. Testicular morphology in intact (top) and pinealectomized (bottom) hamsters killed January 20, 1972, after having been exposed to natural environmental conditions since November 22, 1971. Testicular weight is plotted against body weight for each animal. The height of the bar represents testicular weights for individual hamsters. The shading of the bar indicates whether the testes were histologically atrophic or spermatogenically active. Data from Reiter (1973b).

periods inducing gonadal involution, depressing body weight, and causing the development of white pelage. Characteristically, when animals are maintained under natural photoperiods, they reproduce only between the months of February and November (Figala, Hoffmann, and Goldau, 1973). Their maximum body weight is attained during July and August whereas the minimum occurs in December and January. Molt into the winter coat is induced in summer by exposing the hamsters to short photoperiods (photoperiods normally experienced during the winter). The effects which the light-dark cycle exerts on the reproductive physiology, pelage color,

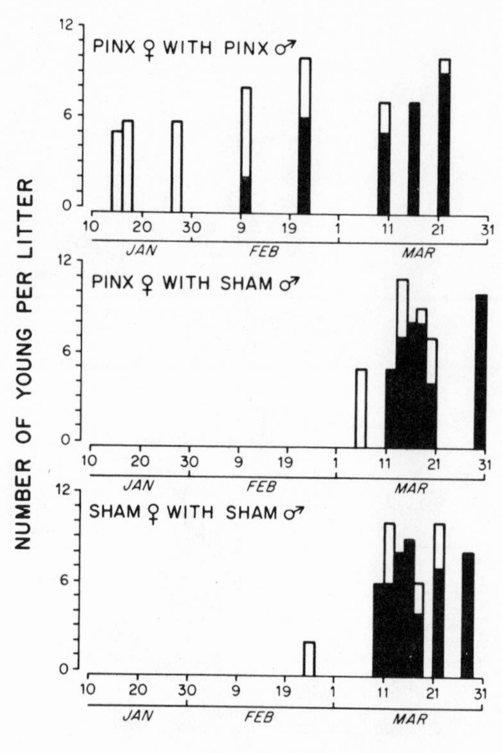

Figure 13. Date of delivery and litter sizes in hamsters kept under natural photoperiodic conditions. Males and females were placed together on December 28. The height of the individual bars represents the sizes of the individual litters. The clear portions of the bars indicate the number of pups that had died or were cannibalized while the dark portion designates the number of animals which survived to weaning (21 days of age). Data from Reiter (1974b).

and body weight are negated in pinealectomized hamsters (K. Hoffmann, personal communication). Thus, the interaction between the photoperiod and the seasonal reproductive cycle seems to be identical with that in the golden hamster (Reiter, 1973a). In the case of the Djungarian hamster, the effects of the pineal on reproduction may somehow be related to melatonin (Hoffmann, 1972; 1973).

The findings of Hoffmann using the Djungarian hamster are very similar to those obtained by Rust and Meyer (1969) who utilized the short-tailed weasel or stoat (Mustela erminea). Normally, this species has a white coat during the winter and a brown coat in summer. Likewise, the gonads atrophy during the short day period of the year (winter). The gonads of summer-captured weasels could be induced to regress if the animals received weekly subcutaneous implants of melatonin in beeswax. Furthermore, these animals molted and grew a white coat. Stoats captured during the winter were already white and were reproductively quiescent. When these animals are exposed to long photoperiods, their reproductive organs recrudesce within a short time and they undergo a pelage color change. Both these processes could be prevented by the subcutaneous implantation of melatonin. Rust and Meyer (1969) interpreted these results to mean that melatonin and presumably the pineal gland plays a significant role in determining seasonal reproductive and pelage color changes in this species.

In another mustelid, the ferret, pineal-gonadal relationships have also been investigated (Herbert, 1971; 1972). Normally, female ferrets kept in natural daylight come into estrus once per year, in the spring. This cycle is apparently very closely regulated since the onset of estrus occurs with great regularity in all animals exposed to the same photoperiod. Likewise, the period of time (about 52 weeks) between the onset of successive estrous periods is very uniform. Light exerts a strong influence on this cycle with photic stimulation during the winter months serving as a stimulus to advance estrous onset. Since the onset of estrus is so closely related to the duration of the daily photoperiod, it seemed likely that the pineal played a role in the synchronization of the cycle.

In view of this, it was anticipated that pinealectomizing ferrets in the fall would lead to an early onset of estrus the following spring. This, however, was not the case (Herbert, 1971; 1972). Ferrets subjected to pinealectomy (in October) during their anestrous period came into estrus at the same time as control ferrets the following spring indicating the possibility that the pineal gland was not essential for estrous onset. Had the experiment been concluded at this time, Herbert could have drawn this conclusion. This is a mistake that has been made by many other investigators. When Herbert (1972) followed the seasonal estrous patterns in his animals for longer periods of time he observed that, in the subsequent spring, the pinealectomized ferrets did not come into estrus at the appropriate time. In fact, ferrets lacking their pineals experienced estrus in the fall, some 20-25 weeks later than normal. Subsequent cycles were similarly prolonged. These data imply that the seasonal reproductive cycle in the ferret may be endogenous with a free-running rhythm of somewhat greater than a year. Photoperiod, acting via the pineal gland, serves to synchronize the cycle with the appropriate season. This is somewhat different than the situation in the hamster where pineal extirpation prevents, in essence, the anestrous period allowing the animals to breed continuously. Although there are obvious basic differences between species, the essential role of the pineal gland in seasonal reproduction seems certain.

V. CONCLUDING REMARKS

If the aforementioned data are considered collectively, it seems that one of the most important functions of the pineal gland may be to synchronize breeding activity in seasonal breeders with the appropriate time of the year. In the absence of this important gland, daylength is unable to exert an influence on reproductive physiology, and either no seasonal rhythm in reproduction occurs (e.g., in hamsters) or the rhythm free runs (e.g., in ferrets). In the latter case the breeding period comes out of phase with the appropriate season of the year.

Whether daily rhythms in endocrine functions are synchronized or impelled by pineal secretions remain, for the most part, unclear. Certainly, the rate of secretion of prolactin during the night seems to depend upon an intact pineal gland. However, the physiological significance of the pineal in influencing daily hormonal fluctuations remains to be determined.

REFERENCES

Albertazzi, E., Barbanti-Silva, C., Trentini, G. P., and Botticelli, A. (1966). Influence de l'epiphysectomie et du traitement avec la 5-hydroxytryptamine sur le cycle oestral de la ratte albinos. Ann. Endocrinol. 27, 93-100.

Allen, C., and Kendall, J. W. (1967). Maturation of the circadian rhythm of plasma corticosterone in the rat. Endocrinology 80, 926-930.

Alleva, J. J., Waleski, M. V., and Alleva, F. R. (1970). The Zeitgeber for ovulation in rats: non-participation of the pineal gland. Life Sci. 9, 241-246.

Axelrod, J., and Weissbach, H. (1960). Enzymatic O-methylation of N-acetylserotonin to melatonin. Science 131, 1312.

Axelrod, J., Wurtman, R. J., and Snyder, S. H. (1965). Control of hydroxyindole-O-methyltransferase activity in the rat pineal gland by environmental lighting. J. Biol. Chem. 240, 949-954.

Benson, B., Matthews, M. J., and Rodin, A. (1971). A melatonin-free extract of bovine pineal with antigonadotropic activity. Life Sci. 10, 607-613.

Benson, B., Matthews, M. J., and Rodin, A. (1972). Studies on a non-melatonin pineal antigonadotropin. Acta Endocrinol. 69, 257-266.

Benson, B., and Orts, R. J. (1972). Regulation of ovarian growth by the pineal gland. In: *Regulation of Organ and Tissue Growth* (Goss, R. J., ed.), pp. 315-335, Academic Press, New York.

Butcher, R. L., Fugo, N. W., and Collins, W. E. (1972). Semicircadian rhythm in plasma levels of prolactin during early gestation in the rat. Endocrinology 90, 1125-1127.

Cardinali, D. P., and Rosner, J. J. (1971). Retinal localization of the hydroxyindole-O-methyltransferase (HIOMT) in the rat. Endocrinology 89, 301-303.

Cardinali, D. P., and Wurtman, R. J. (1972). Hydroxyindole-O-methyltransferase in the rat pineal, retina and Harderian gland. Endocrinology 91, 247-252.

Chazov, Ye. I., Isachenkov, V. A., Krisvosheyev, O. G., Veselova, S. N., and Zhivoderova, G. V. (1972). A factor from the pineal body inhibiting the ovulation induced by luteinizing hormone. Dokl. Acad. Nauk. SSSR, 27, 246-248 (In Russian).
Cheesman, D. W. (1970). Structure elucidation of a gonadotropin inhibiting substance from the bovine pineal gland. Biochim. Biophys. Acta 207, 247-253.
Cheifez, P., Gaffud, N., and Dingman, J. F. (1968). Effects of bilateral adrenalectomy and continuous light on the circadian rhythm of corticotropin in female rats. Endocrinology 82, 1117-1124.
Clark, R. H., and Baker, B. L. (1964). Circadian periodicity in the concentration of prolactin in the rat hypophysis. Science 143, 375-376.
Cuello, A. C., and Tramezzani, J. H. (1969). The epiphysis cerebri of the Weddell seal: its remarkable size and glandular pattern. Gen. Comp. Endocrinol. 12, 154-164.
Donofrio, R. J., and Reiter, R. J. (1972). Depressed pituitary prolactin levels in blinded anosmic female rats: role of the pineal gland. J. Reprod. Fertil. 31, 159-162.
Dunn, J., Dyer, R., and Bennett, M. (1972). Diurnal variation in plasma corticosterone following long term exposure to continuous illumination. Endocrinology 90, 1660-1663.
Dunn, J., Bennett, M., and Peppler, R. (1972). Pituitary-adrenal function in photic and olfactory deprived rats. Proc. Soc. Exptl. Biol. Med. 140, 755-758.
Dunn, J. D., Arimura, A., and Scheving, L. E. (1972). Effect of stress on circadian periodicity in serum LH and prolactin concentration. Endocrinology 90, 29-33.
Ebels, I., Moszkowska, A., and Scemama, A. (1970). An attempt to separate a sheep pineal extract fraction showing antigonadotropic activity. J. Neurovisc. Rel. 32, 1-10.
Elden, C. A., Keyes, M. C., and Marshall, C. E. (1971). Pineal body of the northern fur seal (Callorhinus ursinus): a model for studying the probable function of the mammalian pineal body. Am. J. Vet. Res. 32, 639-647.
Everett, J. W. (1961). The mammalian female reproductive cycle and its controlling mechanisms. In: *Sex and Internal Secretions*, Vol. I, (Young, W. C., ed.), pp. 497-555, Williams and Wilkins, Baltimore.
Figala, J., Hoffmann, K., and Goldau, G. (1973). Zur Jahresperiodik beim Dsungarischen Zwerghamster Phodopus sungorus Pallas. Oecologia 12, 89-118.
Fraschini, F., and Martini, L. (1970). Rhythmic phenomena and pineal principles. In: *The Hypothalamus* (Martini, L., Fraschini, F., and Motta, M., eds.), pp. 529-549, Academic Press, New York.
Freeman, M. E., and Neill, J. D. (1972). The pattern of prolactin secretion during pseudopregnancy in the rat: a daily nocturnal surge. Endocrinology 90, 1291-1294.
Giarman, N. J., Freedman, D. X., and Picard-Ami, L. (1960). Serotonin content of the pineal gland of man and monkey. Nature 186, 480-481.

Hakanson, R., and Owman, C. (1966). Pineal dopa decarboxylase and monoamine oxidase activities as related to monoamine stores. J. Neurochem. 13, 597-605.

Herbert, J. (1971). The role of the pineal gland in the control by light of the reproductive cycle of the ferret. In: *The Pineal Gland* (Wolstenholme, G. E. W. and Knight, J., eds.), pp. 303-327, Churchill Livingstone, London.

Herbert, J. (1972). Initial observations on pinealectomized ferrets kept for long periods in either daylight or artificial illumination. J. Endocrinol. 55, 591-597.

Hiroshige, T., Abe, K., Wada, S., and Kaneko, M. (1973). Sex differences in circadian periodicity of CRF activity in rat hypothalamus. Neuroendocrinology 11, 306-320.

Hoffman, R. A., Hester, R. J., and Towns, C. (1965). Effect of light and temperature on the endocrine system of the golden hamster (Mesocricetus auratus Waterhouse). Comp. Biochem. Physiol. 15, 525-533.

Hoffman, R. A., and Reiter, R. J. (1965). Pineal gland: influence on gonads of male hamsters. Science 148, 1609-1611.

Hoffmann, K. (1972). Melatonin inhibits photoperiodically induced testes development in a dwarf hamster. Naturwissenschaften 59, 218-219.

Hoffmann, K. (1973). The influence of photoperiod and melatonin on testes size, body weight, and pelage colour in the Djungarian hamster (Phodopus sungorus). J. Comp. Physiol. 85, 267-282.

Houssay, A. B., and Barcello, A. C. (1972). Effects of estrogens and progesterone upon the biosynthesis of melatonin by the pineal gland. Experientia 28, 478-479.

Illnerova, H. (1971). Effect of environmental lighting on serotonin rhythm in rat pineal gland during postnatal development. Life Sci. 10, 583-590.

Jacobs, J. J., and Kendall, J. W. (1972). The effect of the pineal on rhythmic pituitary-adrenal function in the blinded rat. Abstracts of Fourth International Congress of Endocrinology, Washington, D.C., p. 53 (Abstract).

Kamberi, I. A., Mical, R. S., and Porter, J. C. (1971). Effects of melatonin and serotonin on the release of FSH and prolactin. Endocrinology 88, 1288-1293.

Klein, D. C., Reiter, R. J., and Weller, J. L. (1971). Pineal N-acetyltransferase activity in blinded and anosmic rats. Endocrinology 89, 1020-1023.

Klein, D. C., and Weller, J. L. (1970). Indole metabolism in the pineal gland: a circadian rhythm in N-acetyltransferase. Science 169, 1093-1095.

Lawton, I. E., and Schwartz, N. B. (1968). A circadian rhythm of luteinizing hormone secretion in ovariectomized rats. Am. J. Physiol. 214, 213-217.

Lerner, A. B., Case, J. D., and Takahashi, Y. (1960). Isolation of melatonin and 5-methoxyindole-3-acetic acid. J. Biol. Chem. 235, 1992-1997.

Lerner, A. B., Case, J. D., Takahashi, Y., Lee, T. H., and Mori, W. (1958). Isolation of melatonin, the pineal gland factor that lightens melanocytes. J. Am. Chem. Soc. 80, 2587.
Longnecker, D. E., and Gallo, D. G. (1971). The inhibition of PMSG-induced ovulation in immature rats by melatonin. Proc. Soc. Exp. Biol. Med. 137, 623-625.
Lynch, H. J. (1971). Diurnal oscillations in pineal melatonin content. Life Sci. 10, 791-795.
Martini, L., Fraschini, F., and Motta, M. (1968). Neural control of the anterior pituitary. Recent Prog. Horm. Res. 24, 439-496.
McGeer, E. G., and McGeer, P. L. (1966). Circadian rhythm in pineal tyrosine hydroxylase. Science 153, 73-74.
McIsaac, W. M., Farrell, G., Taborsky, R. G., and Taylor, A. N. (1965). Indole compounds: isolation from pineal tissue. Science 145, 102-103.
McIsaac, W. M., Taborsky, R. G., and Farrell, G. (1964). 5-methoxytryptophol: effect on estrus and ovarian weight. Science 145, 63-64.
Milcu, S. M., Pavel, S., and Neascu, C. (1963). Biological and chromatographic characterization of a polypeptide with pressor and oxytocic activities isolated from bovine pineal gland. Endocrinology 72, 563-566.
Mogler, R. K.-H. (1958). Das Endokrine System des Syrischen Goldhamster unter Berucksichtizung des Natürlichen und Experimentallen Winterschläf. Z. Morphol. Oekl. Tiere. 47, 167-308.
Morin, L. P. (1973). Ovulatory and body weight response of the hamster to constant light or pinealectomy. Neuroendocrinology 12, 192-198.
Moszkowska, A. (1965). Quelques données nouvelles sur le mecanisme de l'antagonisme épiphyso-hypophysaire. Rôle possible de la sérotonine et de la mélatonine. Rev. Suisse Zool. 72, 145-160.
Moszkowska, A., and Ebels, I. (1971). The influence of the pineal body on the gonadotropic function of the hypophysis. J. Neurovisc. Rel., Suppl. X, 160-176.
Muller, E. E., Guistina, G., Miedico, D., Pecile, A., Cocchi, D., and King, F. W. (1970). Circadian pattern of bioassayable and radioimmunoassayable growth hormone in the pituitary of female rats. Proc. Soc. Exp. Biol. Med. 135, 934-939.
Nesić, Lj. (1962). Contribution a l'etude du rythme saisonnier de la grande pinéale de brebis. Acta Anat. 49, 376-377 (Abstract).
Pavel, S. (1963). Cercetari aspura unui nou hormon pineal cu structura peptidica. Cercet. Endocrinol. 14, 665-668.
Pavel, S. (1971). Evidence for the ependymal origin of arginine vasotocin in the bovine pineal gland. Endocrinology 89, 613-614.
Pavel, S., Petrescu, M., and Vicoleanu, N. (1973). Evidence of central gonadotropin inhibiting activity of arginine vasotocin in the female mouse. Neuroendocrinology 11, 370-374.
Pelham, R. W., and Ralph, C. L. (1972). Diurnal rhythm of serum melatonin in chicken: abolition by pinealectomy. Physiologist 15, 236 (Abstract).
Pelham, R. W., Ralph, C. L., and Campbell, I. M. (1972). Mass spectral identification of melatonin in blood. Biochem. Biophys. Res. Com. 46, 1236-1241.

Pelham, R. W., Vaughan, G. M., Sandock, K. L., and Vaughan, M. K. (1973). Twenty-four hour cycle of a melatonin-like substance in the plasma of human males. J. Clin. Endocrinol. Metab. 37, 341-344.
Pflügfelder, O. (1956). Physiologie der Epiphyse. Deut. Zool. Gesell. Verh. 50, 53-75.
Porter, J. C., Mical, R. S., and Cramer, O. M. (1971/1972). Effect of serotonin and other indoles on the release of LH, FSH and prolactin. Gynecol. Invest., 2, 13-22.
Quay, W. B. (1956). Volumetric and cytologic variation in the pineal body of Peromyscus leucopus (Rodentia) with respect to sex, captivity and day-length. J. Morphol. 98, 471-495.
Quay, W. B. (1963a). Circadian rhythm in rat pineal serotonin and its modifications by estrous cycle and photoperiod. Gen. Comp. Endocrinol. 3, 473-479.
Quay, W. B. (1963b). Differential extraction for the spectrophotofluorometric measurement of diverse 5-hydroxy- and 5-methoxyindoles. Anal. Biochem. 5, 51-59.
Quay, W. B. (1964). Circadian and estrous rhythm in pineal melatonin and 5-hydroxyindole-3-acetic acid. Proc. Soc. Exp. Biol. Med. 115, 710-713.
Quay, W. B., and Halevy, A. (1962). Experimental modification of the rat pineal's content of serotonin and related indoleamines. Physiol. Zool. 35, 1-7.
Ralph, C. L., Mull, D., Lynch, H. J., and Hedlund, L. (1971). A melatonin rhythm persists in rat pineals in darkness. Endocrinology 89, 1361-1366.
Ramaley, J. A. (1973). The development of daily changes in serum corticosterone in pre-weanling rats. Steroids 21, 433-442.
Reiter, R. J. (1968a). The pineal gland and gonadal development in male rats and hamsters. Fertil. Steril. 19, 1009-1017.
Reiter, R. J. (1968b). Pineal-gonadal relationships in male rodents. In: *Progress in Endocrinology* (Gual, C., ed.), pp. 631-636, Excerpta Medica, Amsterdam.
Reiter, R. J. (1969). Pineal function in long term blinded male and female golden hamsters. Gen. Comp. Endocrinol. 12, 460-468.
Reiter, R. J. (1972a). The role of the pineal in reproduction. In: *Reproductive Biology* (Balin, H., and Glasser, S., eds.), pp. 71-114, Excerpta Medica, Amsterdam.
Reiter, R. J. (1972b). Surgical procedures involving the pineal gland which prevent gonadal degeneration in adult male hamsters. Ann. Endocrinol. 33, 571-582.
Reiter, R. J. (1972c). Evidence for refractoriness of the pituitary-gonadal axis to the pineal gland in golden hamsters and its possible implications in annual reproductive rhythms. Anat. Rec. 173, 365-371.
Reiter, R. J. (1973a). Comparative physiology: pineal gland. Ann. Rev. Physiol. 35, 305-328.
Reiter, R. J. (1973b). Pineal control of a seasonal reproductive rhythm in male golden hamsters exposed to natural daylight and temperature. Endocrinology 92, 423-430.

Reiter, R. J. (1974a). Effect of light and the pineal on gonadotropins: some theoretical considerations. In: *Biochemistry and Physiology of the Pineal Gland* (Klein, D. C., ed.), Spectrum Publ. Co., New York, in press.

Reiter, R. J. (1974b). Influence of pinealectomy on the breeding capability of hamsters maintained under natural photoperiodic and temperature conditions. Neuroendocrinology, in press.

Reiter, R. J., and Sorrentino, S., Jr. (1971). Inhibition of luteinizing hormone release and ovulation in PMS-treated rats by peripherally administered melatonin. Contraception 4, 385-392.

Reiter, R. J., Sorrentino, S., Jr., and Ellison, N. M. (1970). Interaction of photic and olfactory stimuli in mediating pineal-induced gonadal regression in adult female rats. Gen. Comp. Endocrinol. 15, 326-333.

Reiter, R. J., Sorrentino, S., Jr., Ralph, C. L., Lynch, H. J., Mull, D., and Jarrow, E. (1971). Some endocrine effects of blinding and anosmia in adult male rats with observations on pineal melatonin. Endocrinology 88, 895-900.

Reiter, R. J., Vaughan, M. K., Vaughan, G. M., Sorrentino, S., Jr., and Donofrio, R. J. (1974). The pineal gland as an organ of internal secretion. In: *Frontiers of Pineal Physiology* (Altschule, M. D., ed.), Harvard University Press, Cambridge, in press.

Rønnekleiv, O. K., Krulich, L., and McCann, S. M. (1973). An early morning surge of prolactin in the male rat and its abolition by pinealectomy. Endocrinology 92, 1339-1342.

Rust, C. C., and Meyer, R. K. (1969). Hair color, molt, and testes size in male, short-tailed weasels treated with melatonin. Science 165, 912-922.

Sassin, J. F., Frantz, A. G., Weitzman, E. D., and Kapen, S. (1972). Human prolactin: 24-hour pattern with increased release during sleep. Science 177, 1205-1207.

Schwartz, N. B. (1970). Control of rhythmic secretion of gonadotropins. In: *The Hypothalamus* (Martini, L., Motta, M., and Fraschini, F., eds.), pp. 515-528, Academic Press, New York.

Schwartz, N. B., and McCormack, C. E. (1972). Reproduction: gonadal function and its regulation. Ann. Rev. Physiol. 34, 425-472.

Simonovic, I., Tima, L., and Martini, L. (1971). "Hypothalamic deafferentation" and gonadotropin secretion. Experientia 27, 211-212.

Smit-Vis, J. H. (1972). The effect of pinealectomy and of testosterone administration on the occurrence of hibernation in adult male golden hamsters. Acta Morph. Neerl. Scand. 10, 269-282.

Smit-Vis, J. H., and Akkerman-Bellaart, M. A. (1967). Spermiogenesis in hibernating golden hamsters. Experientia 23, 844-845.

Snyder, S. H., Axelrod, J., and Zweig, M. (1967). Circadian rhythm in the serotonin content of the rat pineal gland: regulating factors. J. Pharmacol. Exp. Therap. 158, 206-213.

Sorrentino, S., Jr., and Reiter, R. J. (1970). Pineal-induced alteration of estrous cycles in blinded hamsters. Gen. Comp. Endocrinol. 15, 39-42.

Sorrentino, S., Jr., Reiter, R. J., and Schalch, D. S. (1971a). Hypotrophic reproductive organs and normal growth in male rats treated with melatonin. J. Endocrinol. 51, 213-214.

Sorrentino, S., Jr., Schalch, D. S., and Reiter, R. J. (1971b). Environmental control of growth hormone and growth. In: *Growth and Growth Hormone* (Pecile, A., and Muller, E. E., eds.), pp. 330-348, Excerpta Medica, Amsterdam.
Thieblot, L. (1965). Physiology of the pineal body. Prog. Brain Res. 10, 479-488.
Thieblot, L., Alassimare, A., and Blaise, S. (1966). Étude chromatographique et électrophorétique du facteur antigonadotrope de la glande pinéale. Ann. Endocrinol. 27, 861-866.
Thieblot, L., and Blaise, S. (1966). Étude biochimique du principe pinéal antigonadotrope. Probl. Actuels. Endocrinol. Nutr. 10, 257-275.
Thieblot, L., and Menigot, M. (1971). Acquisitions récentes sur le facteur antigonadotrope de la glande pinéale. J. Neurovisc. Rel., Suppl. X, 153-159.
Turner, W. (1888). The pineal body (epiphysis cerebri) in the brain of the walrus and seals. J. Anat. Physiol. 22, 300-303.
Vaughan, M. K., Benson, B., Norris, J. T., and Vaughan, G. M. (1971). Inhibition of compensatory ovarian hypertrophy in mice by melatonin, 5-hydroxytryptamine and pineal powder. J. Endocrinol. 50, 171-175.
Vaughan, M. K., and Klein, D. C. (1973). Effect of arginine vasotocin on gonadal stimulation induced by exogenous or endogenous gonadotrophin. Amer. Zoologist 13, 1288 (Abstract).
Vaughan, M. K., Reiter, R. J., Vaughan, G. M., Bigelow, L., and Altschule, M. D. (1972). Inhibition of compensatory ovarian hypertrophy in the mouse and vole: a comparison of Altschule's pineal extract, pineal indoles, vasopressin and oxytocin. Gen. Comp. Endocrinol. 18, 372-377.
Vlahakes, G., and Wurtman, R. J. (1972). A Mg^{2+} dependent hydroxyindole-O-methyltransferase in the rat Harderian gland. Biochim. Biophys. Acta, 261, 194-198.
Watzka, M., and Voss, H. (1967). Vergleichende histologische Studien an der Zirbel der Vögel. Verh. Anat. Ges. 120, 177-183.
Weiss, B., and Costa, E. (1967). Effect of denervation and environmental lighting on the norepinephrine reduced activation of adenyl cyclase of the rat pineal gland. Fed. Proc. 26, 765 (Abstract).
Weiss, B., and Crayton, J. (1970). Gonadal hormones as regulators of pineal adenyl cyclase activity. Endocrinology 87, 527-533.
Weissbach, H., Redfield, B. G., and Axelrod, J. (1960). Biosynthesis of melatonin: enzymatic conversion of serotonin to N-acetylserotonin. Biochim. Biophys. Acta 43, 352-353.
Wurtman, R. J., and Axelrod, J. (1966). A 24-hour rhythm in the content of norepinephrine in the pineal and salivary glands of the rat. Life Sci. 5, 665-669.
Wurtman, R. J., Axelrod, J., and Chu, E. W. (1963). Melatonin, a pineal substance: effect on the rat ovary. Science 141, 277-278.
Wurtman, R. J., Axelrod, J., and Fischer, J. E. (1964). Melatonin synthesis in the pineal gland: effect of light mediated by the sympathetic nervous system. Science 143, 1329-1330.

Wurtman, R. J., Axelrod, J., and Phillips, L. S. (1963). Melatonin synthesis in the pineal gland: control by light. Science 142, 1071-1072.
Wurtman, R. J., Axelrod, J., Sedvall, G., and Moore, R. Y. (1967). Photic and neural control of the 24-hour norepinephrine rhythm in the rat pineal gland. J. Pharmacol. Exp. Therap. 157, 487-492.
Wurtman, R. J., Axelrod, J., Snyder, S. H., and Chu, W. W. (1965). Changes of the enzymatic synthesis of melatonin in the pineal during the estrous cycle. Endocrinology 76, 798-800.
Ying, S. -Y., and Greep, R. O. (1973). Inhibition of ovulation by melatonin in the cyclic rat. Endocrinology 92, 333-335.
Zieher, L. M., and Pellegrino de Iraldi, A. (1966). Central control of the noradrenaline content in the rat pineal and submaxillary gland. Life Sci. 5, 155-161.

DISCUSSION AFTER DR. REITER'S PAPER

Dr. Ramaley

You showed that plasma melatonin levels in humans (Figure 7) reach a peak at night and pineal melatonin levels in various animals (Figure 6) peak at night. Is there also a peak in the pineal release of melatonin at night in the rat?

Dr. Reiter

The only time melatonin is detected in the blood is at night. It's been looked at, of course, in the human and in the chicken.

Dr. Ramaley

In any animal regardless of diurnal rhythm? My concern is that the human is not generally a nocturnal species and usually the rhythms of human hormones and rat hormones are reciprocal to each other. Yet you showed data suggesting that the melatonin rhythm is the same in both species.

Dr. Reiter

This is the important point. It's been reported that in diurnal species, such as the chicken and the human, HIOMT levels are highest during the daytime and in nocturnal animals they are supposedly highest during the night. Yet when melatonin in the blood or pineal is examined, regardless of whether the animals are diurnal or nocturnal, it is always highest at night. Thus, the melatonin rhythm does not follow the HIOMT rhythm at all.

Dr. Lynch, how would you explain the discrepancy of the elevation in pineal HIOMT in the chicken during the light and yet melatonin appears in the blood during darkness?

Dr. Lynch

It turns out that there is no discrepancy. When we measured chicken pineal melatonin content at intervals around the clock in a flock of chickens that were maintained under diurnal lighting conditions, we were startled to find that in chickens, as in rats, pineal melatonin content is high during the dark phase and low during the light phase of the daily lighting schedule. This was surprising because it appeared to be inconsistent with the report by Lauber et al. (1968), that in chickens the activity of the melatonin forming enzyme, HIOMT, is greater in the light than in darkness. One reason for the apparent discrepancy is, no doubt, the fact that Lauber's observations were made on chickens that had been exposed to constant light or constant darkness for a week and a half and it is clearly unreasonable to extrapolate from the physiological effects of constant conditions to those of diurnal conditions.

The daily variation in pineal HIOMT activity in chickens kept under diurnal lighting conditions has recently been investigated by Pelham and Ralph (1972). They found that when appropriate substrate concentrations were employed in the performance of the enzyme assay, maximum HIOMT activity was observed during the dark phase of the lighting schedule. They further reported that they had failed to demonstrate a rhythmic variation in chicken pineal HIOMT activity when they used the same substrate concentrations as those used by others in the assay of HIOMT activity in the pineals of rats and chickens.

Dr. Reiter

This brings up serious difficulties concerning the early studies on HIOMT rhythms in the pineal. If what you are saying is true, then all the HIOMT studies up until 1970, assuming they used the same assay procedures, are suspect.

Dr. Lynch

The studies of Pelham and Ralph (1972) clearly indicate that at least in its application to the assessment of chicken pineal HIOMT activity, conditions of the assay are critical. Elsewhere, Benjamin Weiss (1968) has shown that the light-induced change of HIOMT activity measured in vitro is related to the concentration of S-adenosylmethionine used in the assay. He suggests that this factor may account for some of the discrepancies that appear in the literature.

Dr. Ramaley

I'm fascinated by your discovery of gonadal regeneration in spite of continuous lighting conditions. Have you explored an explanation for the recurrence of reproductive functions while these animals are still supposedly sleeping in their burrows?

Dr. Reiter

The spontaneous regeneration of the gonads is the most exciting part of the circannual rhythm in the hamster. It's difficult to explore until we know what the pineal hormone is in the case of the hamster. Is it melatonin? Is it methoxytryptophol? Is it a polypeptide or is it some other indole? Until we know that, there is nothing we can adequately measure in the pineal gland to determine if it is being shut down during the period of gonadal regeneration. I do not know what accounts for the spontaneous regeneration. Something either inhibits the pineal gland or possibly the system becomes refractory to the pineal influence. In the case of the hamster, we have repeatedly given melatonin under a wide variety of conditions and never shown it to have any effect on the reproductive system. This does not categorically mean that melatonin is not the hormone in the hamster. We may be testing it under inappropriate conditions. It's suggestive that it is not very important in the hamster. But whether it is not the hormone, I am not prepared to say.

Dr. Kitay

My question has to do with the fact that in the studies you've presented about hamster testicular function, so far as I can make out, you have testicular weight and reproductive capability as parameters of testicular function. Now, the testes have two functions as you know, one of which is reproductive and the other hormonal. Can you make any definitive comment concerning the effect of your manipulations on Leydig cell function and testosterone secretion?

Dr. Reiter

We have not measured testosterone. On the basis of the atrophic accessory sex organs, which I didn't go into, we feel that both LH and testosterone are depressed. So presumably the Leydig cells are inhibited due to the depressed LH levels. In addition, there may be some direct effects of the pineal on the gonads. There is evidence, for example, that melatonin interferes with the synthesis of androgens within the testes (Peat and Kinson, 1971). Whether this is the normal function of melatonin, I don't know. These studies were done using tissue culture.

Dr. Krieger

With regard to your statement that melatonin had no effect on hibernating animals, I wonder if there are any endogenous changes in melatonin, arginine vasotocin or the methoxytryptophols in pineals of hibernating animals.

Dr. Reiter

No one has ever looked at the biochemistry of pineal glands from animals killed during hibernation. I will give you one bit of information that may say something about the role of melatonin. Presumably there is a melatonin rhythm within the pineal gland. If that is true, and if melatonin is the antigonadotrophic substance, pineals taken from night-killed animals should be more antigonadotrophic than pineals taken from day-killed animals. When injected into assay animals, there is no appreciable difference in the antigonadotrophic potential of pineals of day- or night-killed rats. We have not assessed the antigonadotrophic capabilities of animals killed during hibernation.

Dr. Krieger

The data on the hibernating animals are very suggestive as you say, for a pineal role in holding. In a nonseasonal breeder, like a human, what would you think the function of the pineal is?

Dr. Reiter

First of all, there are studies that come from northern Finland which show that, in fact, conception rate is significantly higher during the summer months than during the winter months (Timonen et al., 1964). Many of the individuals studied in this particular case were Laplanders living within the Arctic Circle where they experienced long winter nights and long summer days. In these individuals there was a seasonal rhythm in reproduction, particularly noticeable when you look at multiple conceptions, i.e., twins and triplets. The function of the pineal gland in the human is a little difficult to assess at this early date. In view of the basic effect of the pineal gland on biogenic amines within the brain, it may be related to sleep, to periodic psychoses, and to psychoses generally, such as schizophrenia. Undoubtedly, pineal tumors are related to precocious puberty and delayed pubescense.

Dr. Krieger

The data you gave on prolactin, I thought, were extremely interesting. You mentioned that the level of prolactin within the pituitary was decreased. Does this represent decreased synthesis or increased release, and what happens to prolactin levels in the peripheral blood?

Dr. Reiter

I'm glad you asked that question. We would have predicted elevated levels of prolactin in the blood. After long-term light deprivation there is no detectable elevation in plasma prolactin levels. We have not looked at the early response to light deprivation. I would predict that immediately after dark exposure prolactin levels go up in the plasma. Possibly, the hypersecretion of prolactin eventually exhausts the pituitary of its supply and as a result, after long-term light deprivation, plasma prolactin levels drop. We are in the process of testing this possibility.

Dr. Prahlad

In your 1969 review you stated that nobody has studied the effects of different spectrums of light on the pineal. Has anybody done any work on this problem since then?

Dr. Reiter

I haven't but Dr. Lynch's group has. I don't know if he's going to discuss that today. There are several published reports, one by Cardinali et al. (1972) and one by Vriend and Lauber (1973).

Dr. Hedlund.

Is there any relationship between pineal activity and TSH and TRH levels?

Dr. Reiter

We have never measured TSH in animals with stimulated pineals. I think the pineal gland has effects on the entire neuroendocrine axis, including TSH. We know, e.g., that it affects growth hormone, gonadotrophins, and prolactin. Specifically, with regards to your question, I don't know; we have not looked at TRH or TSH levels.

Dr. Prahlad

What is the level of prolactin in hibernating animals?

Dr. Reiter

I will tell you in roughly three weeks. The experiments are in progress.

Dr. Karsch

I was particularly intrigued by the experiments you described in ferrets and if I interpreted them correctly, the effect of pinealectomy on the breeding season is not seen for several years. If the pineal gland is a controller of the breeding season phenomenon, why does seasonal breeding persist for a year or two in the absence of the pineal?

Dr. Reiter

First of all, I think it was actually very fortuitous that Herbert found that estrus in the pinealectomized ferret was not delayed the first year. Had that been so, the criticism would have been that the severe surgical procedure (pinealectomy) delayed the onset of estrus the first year. Obviously, somehow the system is programmed far in advance, at least prior to the previous October when the pinealectomies were done. Dr. Halberg, I know relatively little about the programming of cycles. I presume this is something that is a possibility.

Dr. Halberg

I would guess it matters little whether estrus "arrives in time" and then delays, or "arrives in time" and then advances. Professor Sundararaj has shown that in continuous light, for instance, the catfish may show no change in timing of ovarian recrudescence in the first year, whereas the increase in ovarian weight may advance during the second and third years, this advance in continuous light being more pronounced than that in continuous darkness. Since light and darkness no longer provide a time cue under either of these two conditions, and since temperature is rigidly controlled, one must indeed assume, as you point out, Russ, that circannual rhythms in this species are pre-programmed.

It will be very important indeed to look at these possibilities of pre-programming or of genetic coding of rhythms in the case of circannual changes since today we confront skeptics who believe that circannual rhythms are all impressed from without and persisting from within, a status reminiscent of what was the general view held with respect to circadian rhythms in the 1950's.

I did wish to present to you a well-deserved bouquet for the most interesting ground you have covered in your presentation. Indeed you discussed many circannual phenomena. Let me add that the evidence is now overwhelming for another set of circannual rhythms, namely those in norepinephrine and epinephrine excretion. In our hands these are some of the most prominent circannual phenomena. Dr. Julius Axelrod has pointed out that the driving factor for many of these catecholamine excretion rhythms may well be the rhythms in brain amines.

DISCUSSION REFERENCES

Cardinali, D., Larin, F., and Wurtman, R. J. (1972). Proc. Natl. Acad. Sci. USA 69, 2003-2005.
Lauber, J., Boyd, J., and Axelrod, J. (1968). Science 161, 489-490.
Peat, F., and Kinson, G. A. (1971). Steroids 17, 251-264.
Pelham, R., and Ralph, C. (1972). Life Sci. 11, 51-59.
Timonens, S., Franzas, B., and Wichmann, K. (1964). Ann. Chir. Gynaec. Fenn. 53, 165-172.
Vriend, J., and Lauber, J. K. (1973). Nature 244, 37-38.
Weiss, B. (1968). Adv. Pharmacol. 6A, 152-155.

AN ANALYSIS OF THE PINEAL HYDROXYINDOLE-O-METHYL TRANSFERASE RHYTHM DURING THE ESTROUS CYCLE OF THE RAT

E. P. Wallen and J. M. Yochim

Department of Physiology and Cell Biology
University of Kansas
Lawrence, Kansas 66044

For the past few years our laboratory has been interested in the relationship between pineal gland rhythmicity and reproductive function in the rat. As an index of pineal rhythmicity we followed the diurnal variations in hydroxyindole-O-methyl transferase (HIOMT), the enzyme which forms melatonin, one of the pineal's antigonadotropic hormones. We have interpreted the effects of endocrine and environmental manipulation in terms of changes in a mixed-wave equation.

Our first experiment was to measure the daily fluctuations in HIOMT during the estrous cycle of the rat; from these data we derived the mixed-wave equation (Wallen and Yochim, 1973a). On the ordinate of Figure 1 is enzyme activity in picomoles of [^{14}C]melatonin formed/hr/gland as a function of the 4-day estrous cycle and the first six days of pseudopregnancy. Enzyme activity was measured at least three times daily, six rats per point, according to a modified method of the procedure of Axelrod, Wurtman and Snyder (1965). The sinusoidal curves shown below the enzyme activity represent the postulated 24-hour and 20-hour (or 19.2 hour) rhythms which sum to give the generated upper pattern. It s evident that this pattern matches closely the empirically derived points as represented by solid circles plus or minus the standard error of the mean. A "beat-period" occurs during the estrous-metestrous period and it occurs when the two component rhythms oppose each other (Halberg, 1960). In general, enzyme activity peaks during the dark, and troughs in the light. It is to be noted also that the periods of maximal fluctuations coincide with periods of increased vaginal cornification, while low cornification is found during the low amplitudes of the "beat period" or pseudopregnancy. Analysis of variance followed by a test of the least significant difference between the means indicated that the oscillations during all stages of the cycle except the "beat period" were significantly different ($P < .05$).

This work was supported by USPHS Grant HD0416 and by NICHHD Research Career Development Award 1 K04-HD8558 to J.M.Y.

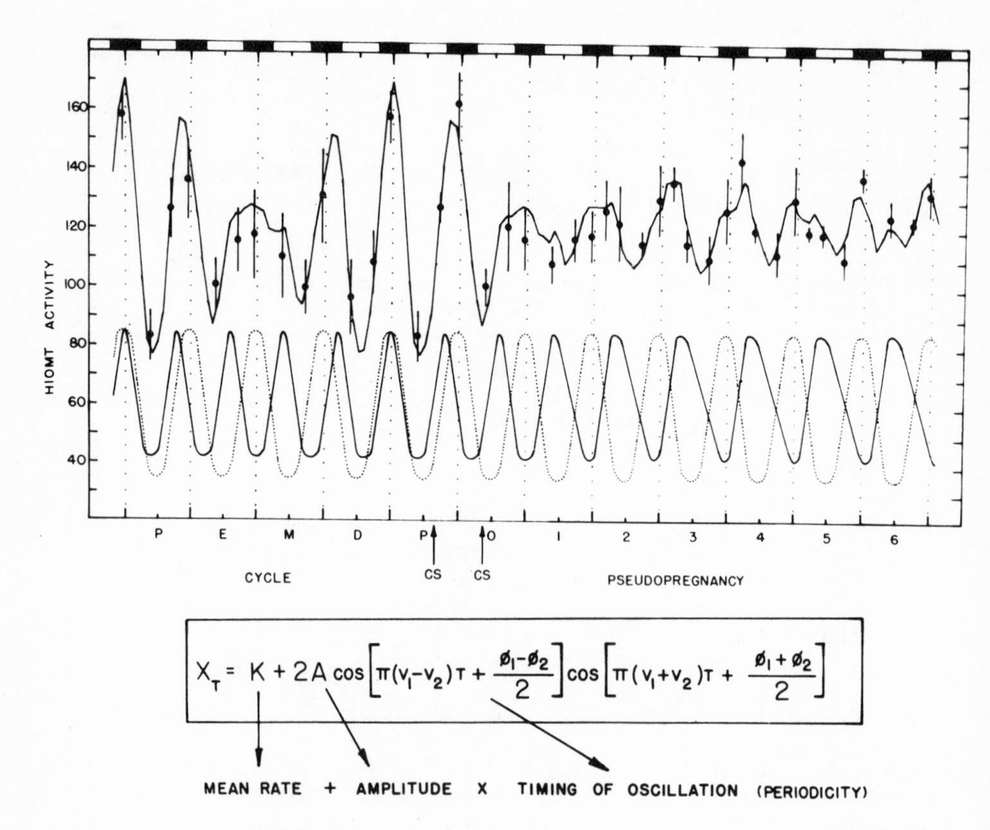

Figure 1. Hydroxyindole-O-methyltransferase (HIOMT) activity during the 4-day estrous cycle and the first six days of pseudopregnancy in the rat. The lower curves represent the component, hypothetical rhythms which add to give the resultant, upper curve. The solid, lower curve exhibits a rhythm of 19.2 hours during the 4-day cycle (20 hours during a 50-day cycle). This rhythm shifts to 24.8 hours following cervical stimulation (CS). The dotted, lower curve is related to the light-dark rhythm (24 hours). The upper curve, which is the sum of these component rhythms, matches the data depicted by the points ± standard error of the mean (N = 6 rats/point). On the lower portion of this figure is the equation which generates HIOMT activity (X_T) based on the interaction of two sine waves whose amplitudes, periods and phase relations are similar to the component rhythms in Figure 1.

On the rightehand portion of Figure 1 it is to be noted that following the induction of pseudopregnancy by cervical stimulation, the pattern of HIOMT changes immediately and can be accounted for by a slight delay in the declining leg of the 20-hour component (Yochim and Wallen, 1973a). This component changes its periodicity from 20 hours as found during the estrous cycle, to 24.8 hours. Thus, induction of pseudopregnancy alters one of the periodicity terms of the equation.

On the lower portion of Figure 1 is the general equation for the interaction of two component rhythms with slightly different frequencies. In this equation HIOMT activity (X_T) is the result of 3 terms: mean rate (K), amplitude (A) and periodicity (V). In all subsequent studies the variations in HIOMT activity will be discussed as a modification in one or more of the three major terms of this equation.

The next series of experiments was designed to test the effects of continuous light (CL) or continuous darkness (CD) on HIOMT activity (Yochim and Wallen, 1973b). On the left portion of Figure 2 is the

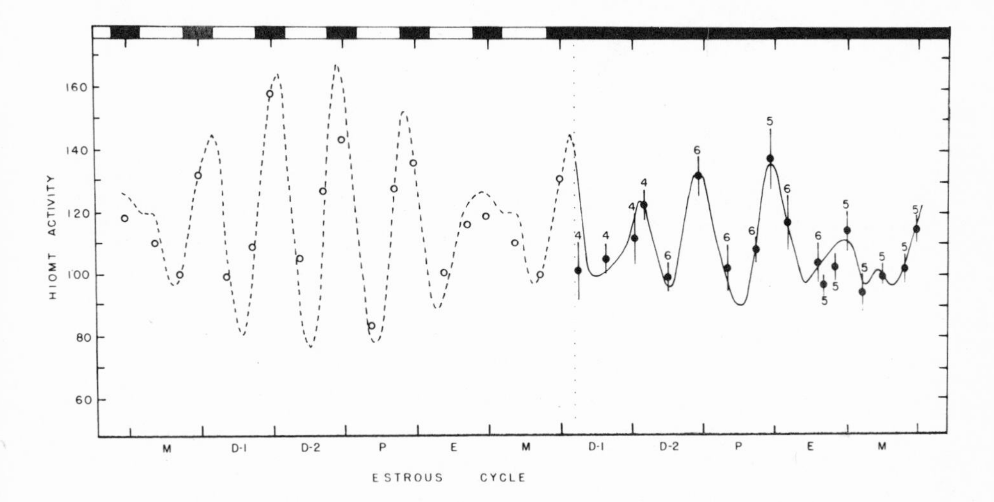

Figure 2. Effect of continuous darkness on HIOMT activity during the estrous cycle. Dashed curve is the pattern of enzyme activity from the 5-day estrous cycle (Yochim and Wallen, 1973b). The solid curve represents HIOMT activity during 5 days exposure to continuous darkness. (Number of rats is listed above each S.E.M.)

normal 5-day estrous cycle pattern. When rats were placed into CD beginning on metestrus, the periodicity was maintained while the mean rate and amplitude decreased only slightly. To our knowledge this is the first demonstration of the persistence of a HIOMT rhythm among female rats in CD. It is evidenced only if rats are synchronized according to estrous cycle stage. In contrast to these results, when rats were placed into CL, all rhythmicity was soon lost and there was a gradually cascading mean rate of enzyme activity (Yochim and Wallen, 1973b).

In Figure 3 we present the effects of altering the proportion of light per day on the mean rate and amplitude of enzyme activity. Both

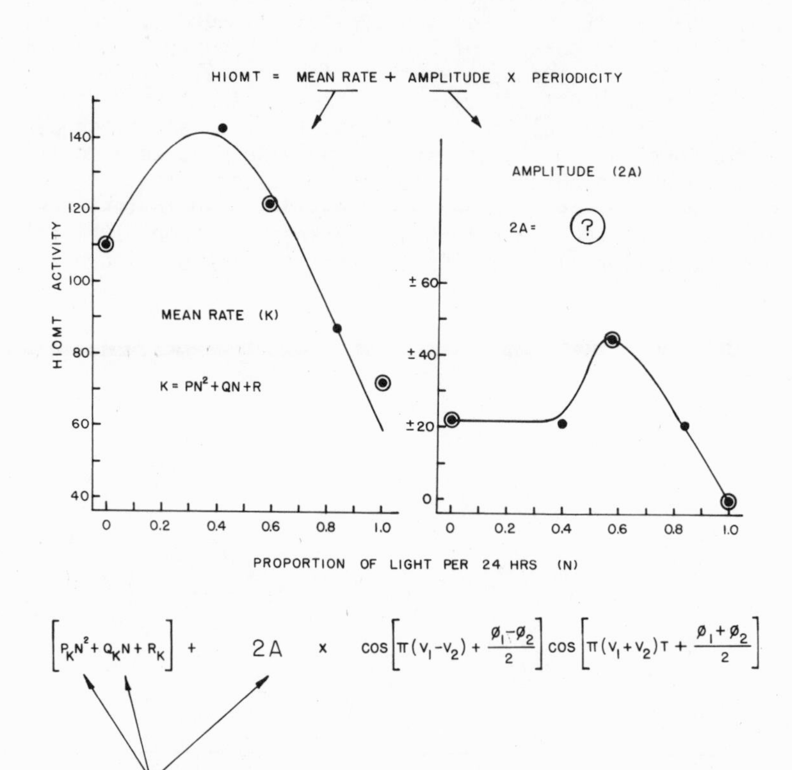

$$\left[P_K N^2 + Q_K N + R_K\right] + 2A \times \cos\left[\pi(v_1 - v_2) + \frac{\phi_1 - \phi_2}{2}\right] \cos\left[\pi(v_1 + v_2)T + \frac{\phi_1 + \phi_2}{2}\right]$$

Figure 3. Effects of proportion of light per day (N) on mean rate (K) and amplitude (A) of HIOMT activity. The mean rate of enzyme activity varies parabolically with the changes in proportion of light per day. Circled points indicate data collected during a complete cycle. No estimate of variability is presented since K and A are derived secondarily from the raw data. On the lower portion of this figure is a summary of the effect of the proportion of light on the terms in the HIOMT mixed-wave equation. The mean rate (K) term is presented in its expanded form to indicate which terms in the quadratic are affected by the proportion of light.

the mean rate and amplitude are plotted as a function of the proportion of light in a 24-hour period. For the mean rate, the response was parabolic, which allowed expansion of this term as shown in Figure 3. This expanded equation demonstrates that light is having an effect on two terms in the parabolic equation. No attempt was made to do a similar analysis on the amplitude term due to its more complex nature.

The last experiment to be discussed involved the effects of ovarian hormones on HIOMT activity (Wallen and Yochim, 1973b). Following ovariectomy on the morning of metestrus, as shown on Figure 4, it can be seen

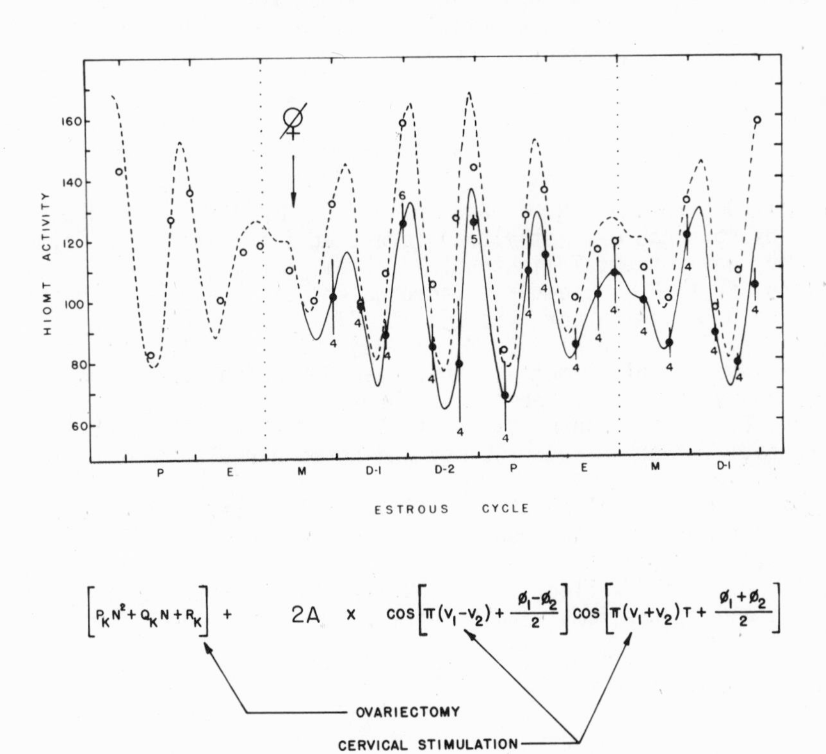

$$\left[P_K N^2 + Q_K N + R_K\right] + 2A \times \cos\left[\pi(v_1 - v_2) + \frac{\phi_1 - \phi_2}{2}\right] \cos\left[\pi(v_1 + v_2)T + \frac{\phi_1 + \phi_2}{2}\right]$$

Figure 4. Changes in HIOMT activity following ovariectomy during metestrus of the estrous cycle. The upper curve (dotted line) is the pattern of enzyme activity found in intact rats during the 5-day cycle while the lower pattern (solid line) represents the daily changes in HIOMT activity for 6 days following ovariectomy. The number of animals is shown above or below each standard error of the mean. Below the graph is a summary of the effect of ovarian hormones and neural cues on the terms in the HIOMT mixed-wave equation.

that there is a significant decrease in the mean rate (K) from 120 to 100 picomoles of [^{14}C]melatonin formed while the periodicity is maintained. A similar effect occurred following ovariectomy and the induction of pseudopregnancy. It is important to note that while these rats have been ovariectomized, they continue to exhibit an "estrous cycle pattern" (Fig. 4).

In summary, the experiments discussed demonstrate that HIOMT activity in the female rat is a reflection of a mixed-wave equation whose mean rate (K) is regulated by ovarian hormones and the proportion of light per day and whose periodicity is affected by neural cues such as copulation or cervical stimulation.

REFERENCES

Axelrod, J., Wurtman, R. J. and Snyder, S. H. (1965). Control of hydroxyindole-O-methyltransferase activity in the rat pineal gland by environmental lighting. J. Biol. Chem. 240, 949-954.

Halberg, F. (1960). Temporal coordination of physiologic function. Cold Spring Harbor Symp. Quant. Biol. 25, 289-310.

Wallen, E. P. and Yochim, J. M. (1973a). Rhythmic function of pineal hydroxyindole-O-methyltransferase during the estrous cycle: an analysis. Biol. Reprod. In press.

Wallen, E. P. and Yochim, J. M. (1973b). Pineal HIOMT activity in the rat: effect of ovariectomy and hormone replacement. Biol. Reprod. In press.

Yochim, J. M. and Wallen, E. P. (1973a). Function of the pineal gland of the rat during progestation: alterations in HIOMT rhythmicity. Biol. Reprod. In press.

Yochim, J. M. and Wallen, E. P. (1973b). HIOMT activity in the pineal gland of the female rat: effects of light. Biol. Reprod. In press.

CORRELATION BETWEEN HYDROXYINDOLE-O-METHYL TRANSFERASE RHYTHMICITY AND REPRODUCTIVE FUNCTION IN THE RAT

J. M. Yochim and E. P. Wallen

Department of Physiology and Cell Biology
University of Kansas
Lawrence, Kansas 66044

INTRODUCTION

Dr. Wallen has presented a simplified mathematical model of hydroxy-indole-O-methyltransferase (HIOMT) activity which can account for physiological changes in enzyme activity imposed by (a) the presence or absence of ovarian hormones, (b) the application of neuroendocrine stimuli such as the induction of pseudopregnancy, and (c) a change in the proportion of light per day (Wallen and Yochim, 1973a,b; Yochim and Wallen, 1973a,b). These effects could be simulated by changing the numerical value of one or more terms on a mixed-wave equation.

However, to test the validity of the mixed-wave equation as a model, it was necessary to determine its response to alterations in photoperiod, i.e., changes in the duration of the daily rhythm. We tested this by modifying the phase relation between the two rhythmic components of the equation, as described in Figure 1 (Wallen and Yochim, 1973c; Yochim and Wallen, 1973c).

In the upper portion of Figure 1 is depicted the characteristic estrous cycle pattern of HIOMT activity. This pattern is a reflection of the interaction of a hypothetical light-cued 24-hour component with a hypothetical, endogenous 20-hour component. When the components are in phase, large amplitudes are observed. These occur during periods of increased estrogen secretion (late diestrus-proestrus). Conversely, when the hypothetical components are out of phase, a beat period with depressed amplitude is observed. This phenomenon is associated with periods of decreased estrogen secretion (metestrus). Our experimental design was to decrease the period of the 24-hour component to 20 hours by changing the photoperiod while retaining the same light:dark (L:D) relationship (14L:10D changed to 11.67L:8.33D).

This work was supported by USPHS Grant HD04016 and by NICHHD Research Career Development Award 1 K04-HD8558 to J.M.Y.

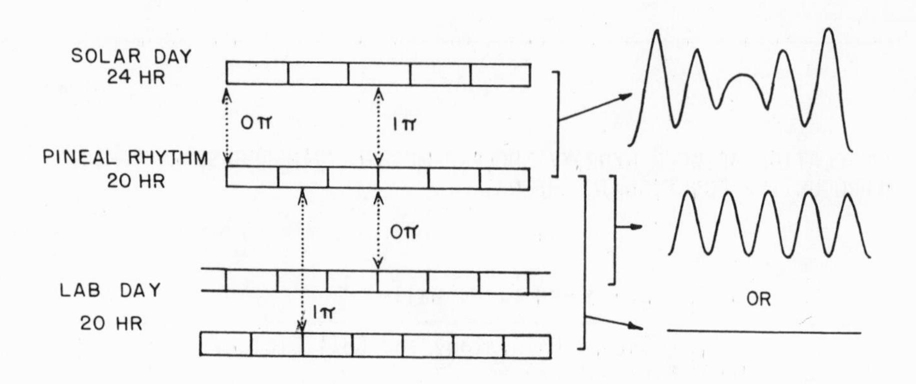

Figure 1. Representation of the interactions between hypothetical 24-hour and 20-hour rhythms during a five day solar period (upper curve) or between two 20-hour rhythms during the same period (lower curves). The change in the HIOMT activity rhythm of rats exposed to the 20-hour environment should depend on the phase relationship between the two component rhythms.

The equation indicates that if rats are exposed to the new environment such that the endogenous rhythm is in phase with the photoperiod, then HIOMT activity should oscillate with constant amplitudes and no beat period. Conversely, if rats are exposed to the new environment such that the endogenous rhythm is out of phase with the environment, HIOMT should not oscillate (lower portion of Figure 1). We did this experiment as follows. Following exposure of rats for about 12 days to the 20-hour environment such that the endogenous rhythm was in phase with the photoperiod, large amplitudes in HIOMT activity were measured (Figure 2, left). Peak activity was measured during the dark, with troughs occurring during the light. Conversely, animals exposed to the environment such that the hypothetical pineal component was out of phase with the photoperiod showed no significant oscillation in HIOMT activity (Figure 2, right). Since all animals were exposed to the same photoperiod for the same duration of time under identical conditions, we concluded that the difference in response of the two groups was a reflection of the phase elationship between the pineal 20-hour component and the photoperiod-cued 20-hour component.

Biological confirmation of the relationship between HIOMT activity and reproductive function was obtained following exposure of rats to the experimental environment for 20 days under conditions selected to generate specific phase relationships between the pineal component and the environment. Animals exposed such that the rhythms were in phase (0.2π radians) showed a significantly higher incidence of vaginal cornification than those exposed such that the rhythmic components were out

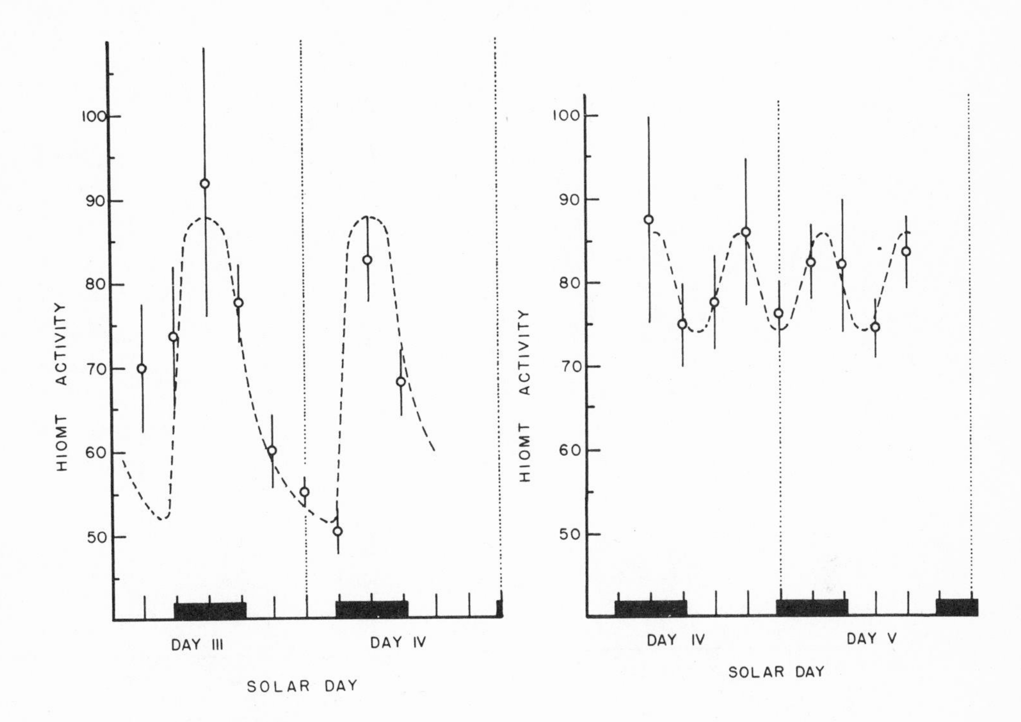

Figure 2. HIOMT activity (pmoles/hour/gland ± SEM) in rats exposed to a 20 hour photoperiod for about 12 days such that an endogenous component was in phase (left) or out of phase (right) with the photoperiod.

of phase (1.0-1.4π radians). Pinealectomy abolished the difference between these groups (Figure 3). The details of experimental design are presented elsewhere (Wallen and Yochim, 1973c; Yochim and Wallen, 1973c).

These results, along with those presented by Dr. Wallen (this volume), can be summarized in a block-diagram as shown in Figure 4. Five major components are shown: ovary, pituitary gland, hypothalamus, pineal gland and a postulated "rhythm perception area" which we have depicted as anatomically separate from the hypothalamus, but which need not be. We suggest that this perception area generates the basic rhythm, which is modified by the various parameters we have measured listed at the top of the diagram as "cues". The modified rhythm is transmitted simultaneously to the pineal gland and to the hypothalamus; thus, pinealectomy does not abolish the basic rhythm. The pineal gland transduces this "information" into a rhythmic change in antigonadotropic secretory activity, which we have monitored as HIOMT activity, modifying the function of the hypothalamo-hypophyseal-gonadal axis. Feedback information from the gonad affects the rhythm perception area as diagrammed.

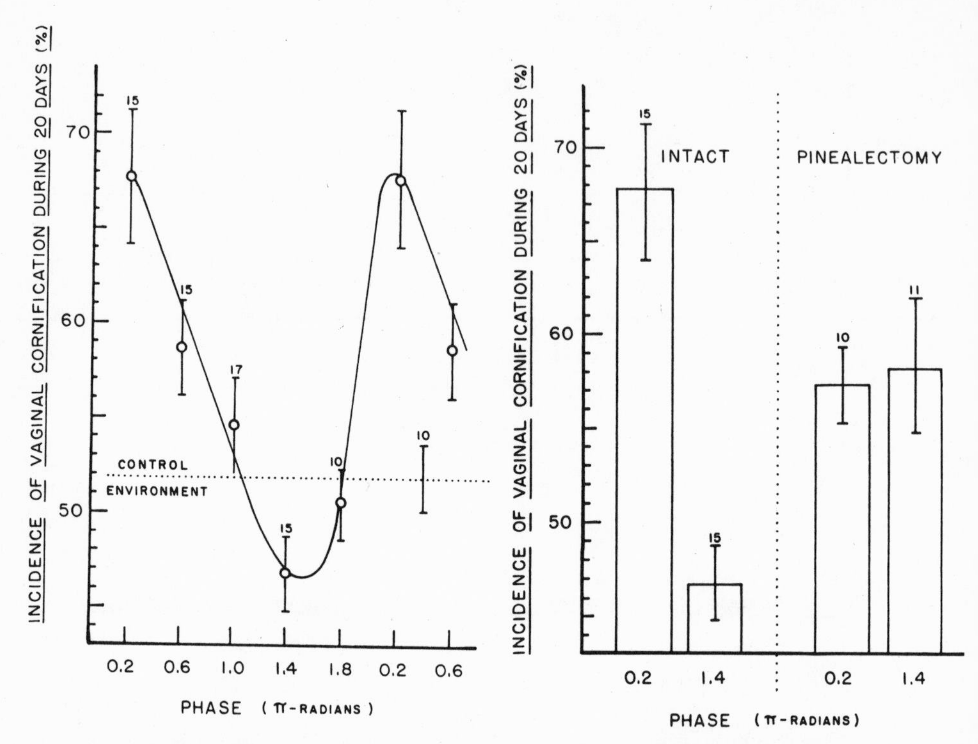

Figure 3. Effect of the 20-hour photoperiod on the incidence of vaginal cornification in intact (left) and pinealectomized (right) rats. The values (mean ± S.E.M.) are plotted according to the hypothetical phase relationship between the pineal 20-hour component and the 20-hour photoperiod.

Whether or not this model will prove useful in the study of other animals remains to be examined. However, it appears to be a reasonable representation of the relationship between light, pineal function and reproductive activity in the rat.

REFERENCES

Wallen, E. P. and Yochim, J. M. (1973a). Rhythmic function of pineal hydroxyindole-O-methyl transferase during the estrous cycle: an analysis. Biology of Reproduction. In press.

Wallen, E. P. and Yochim, J. M. (1973b). Pineal HIOMT activity in the rat: effect of ovariectomy and hormone replacement. Biology of Reproduction. In press.

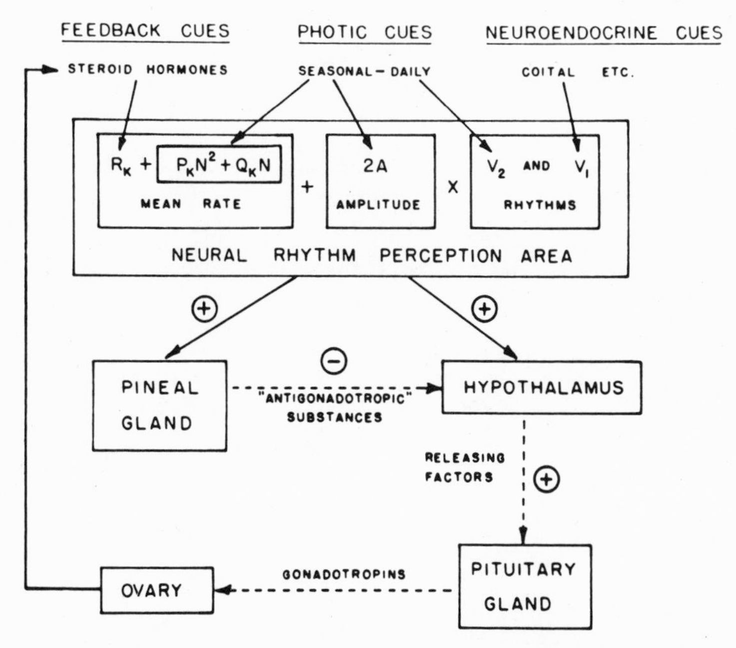

Figure 4. Relationship between pineal function and reproductive neuro-endocrinology in the rat. Solid arrows indicate those relationships examined directly or indirectly by the authors. Dashed arrows connect a highly simplified framework of the basic neuroendocrine unit involved in reproductive function. A = amplitude; P,Q,R = empirically determined constants; N = proportion of light per day; V_1 and V_2 represent two endogenous rhythmic components; + and - symbols indicate the major effects, whether positive or negative (Yochim and Wallen, 1973c).

Wallen, E. P. and Yochim, J. M. (1973c). Photoperiodic regulation of the estrous cycle of the rat: role of the pineal gland. Biology of Reproduction. In press.

Yochim, J. M. and Wallen, E. P. (1973a). HIOMT activity in the pineal gland of the female rat: effects of light. Biol. Reprod. In press.

Yochim, J. M. and Wallen, E. P. (1973b). Function of the pineal gland of the rat during progestation: alterations in HIOMT rhythmicity. Biol. Reprod. In press.

Yochim, J. M. and Wallen, E. P. (1973c). Photoperiod, pineal HIOMT activity and reproductive function in the rat: a proposed model. Biol. Reprod. In press.

DISCUSSION AFTER DR. WALLEN'S AND DR. YOCHIM'S PAPERS

Dr. Halberg

Does your model require that the two components have identical amplitudes?

Dr. Yochim

No, it does not. We did this for simplicity.

Dr. Halberg

If I do a mental cosine fit on Figure 2 (Yochim and Wallen), I would say that on the right the fit of the cosine is almost as good as on the left. This impression in no way detracts from your model; you would have to have a straight line in the cancellation only if the two components were not only "out-of-phase" but would also have identical amplitudes. You still should be congratulated for these results, whether or not you modify the theoretical prediction on Figure 1 (Yochim and Wallen) where you say that either amplification or total cancellation may result.

Dr. Yochim

Yes, you are right. The predictions on Figure 1 (Yochim and Wallen) show only the extreme conditions under the assumption of equal amplitudes. A damping would occur if the amplitudes were not identical.

Dr. Kitay

I have a question that really doesn't arise specifically from these data. It has to do with what criteria one uses for evaluating the validity of the assumption of rhythm in data. I am reminded about an article that was written in Science some years ago concerning the derivation of biological rhythms in a unicorn (Cole, 1957) and has to do with the fact that one can, with appropriate mathematical manipulation, introduce recurring cyclic patterns in data which had no intrinsic cyclic variability. I don't know of anything other than a kind of retrospective seat-of-the-pants judgement that determines whether one fits a straight line, a cosine curve, or parabolic curve, or whatever, to data. The choice seems to depend on criteria which, so far as I know, has yet to be presented with a means of evaluating the validity or the chances of error in such curve fitting.

Dr. Yochim

I don't quite know how other people do this and we're rather new at it, but what we did was to fit these curves as best we could to test as a model. Now, if the experimental evidence showed that the equations wouldn't work then, of course, we would drop the model. As it turned out, they seemed to fit fairly well and so we had no reason to drop the model just yet.

Dr. Kitay

I didn't mean to question that. It seems to me though, that in any set of data that there are many interpretations that are possible. There is an infinite family of curves that could be fitted. You happen to have chosen one that did fit. My question has to do with what objective criteria do we employ to evaluate the validity of the curve that fits. Is the decision determined by future experiments or is it an esthetic judgement?

Dr. Wallen

At the basis of our analysis is the observation of "beats" and I think Dr. Halberg will support me if I say that this is something which is strictly observed and it can only be initially discerned from an observation of the data.

Dr. Halberg

Let me agree with Dr. Kitay that a good analysis requires test criteria -- statistical, and what is even more important, testable biologic assumptions. From both viewpoints you may include an error term in your model. You just take the very nice equation you have and add an error term and then test for zero amplitude. This is acceptable if a period can be anticipated from biologic observations at low noise levels, and thereby one distinguishes the unicorn from the non-unicorn.

Certain rhythms are quite prominent. A so-called spike-dome stands out in the electroencephalogram. It repeats itself with sufficient prominence so that a zero-amplitude test is superfluous for the very recognition of the condition. The same may apply for paroxysmal discharge in the electroencephalogram. By the same token, an experienced electrocardiographer may recognize a coronary from his tracing with the naked eye -- in about 50% of his cases. In another 50% of the cases with coronary infarction, however, he may miss the event if he relies solely on the electrocardiogram. The question of subjectivity and objectivity in biology and medicine is a much discussed one. I am inclined to take the view of the conservative unbeliever and would insist that even for certain studies of the electroencephalogram (Crowley et al., 1972) that amplitude tests or similar procedures be carried out.

Dr. Yochim

I guess I must have misunderstood. We analyzed this, that is, visually at first, but we did do an analysis of variance on the entire equation and determined that the peaks and troughs in the equation were significant except for the "beat period" where there was no significant amplitude generated. Now, perhaps this answers the question.

Dr. Halberg

If the model, whoever's model, allows one to predict the outcome of an otherwise confusing situation in say 95%, if not 100% of the cases, this result should be acceptable. It is a much better result than the evidence for many a diagnosis in medicine. Many of our tests currently in clinical use may have a much more modest measure of predictability. By contrast, the occurrence of circadian periods (non-24-hour [desynchronized] or synchronized and perhaps both) has now been amply documented. Actually, some free-running periods, as in the blinded C-mouse, are so predictable that the knowledge of an antiphase with respect to controls, say during the end of the third week after blinding, allows verification of desynchronization with a single sample from a blinded animal as compared to a single sample from a control. Actually, data from the early 1950's on desynchronization of the rectal temperature rhythm after blinding were confirmed or extended not only by separate investigators in Minnesota but also by investigators who were using the Minnesota animals at the Ames Research Center of NASA in Mountain View, California.

There will come a time when a discussion of circadian rhythms will be dissociated from the matter of artifacts, just as eventually people realized that there was a circulation even though they kept on using reference to arteries. Most of us may remember that arteries were so named because air was assumed to flow through them. Malaria was designated as a disease brought about by "bad air." Some "rhythms" indeed are artifacts, notably when they are assessed by endocrinologists who choose to ignore, in 1974, that the chances of a high corticoid value in human blood will be different in the morning and in the evening, respectively.

Let me once more indicate that biologic evidence in "noise-reduced" situations on the mechanisms of rhythms, obtained by first standardizing conditions and then using the time-honored approach of "remove and replace" is essential. However, once "clean" data have led to the discovery of entities such as the adrenal cycle, it seems useful to develop methods whereby in a "noisy" field situation the characteristics of rhythms can be defined, and what is more important, quantified in health and disease, e.g., by the fit of a cosine or preferably of several cosines. By fitting such cosines, as one of many possible approaches, one no more claims that the cosine fit represents the rhythm than one claims that a microscope models the cell. In both cases one resolves a phenomenon on hand without taking the resolving tool as a model for the biologic entity.

DISCUSSION REFERENCES

Cole, L. C. (1957). Science 125, 874-876.

Crowley, T., Kripke, D., Halberg, F., Pegram, G., and Schildkraut, J. (1972). Primates 13, 149-168.

SYMPATHETIC NEURAL CONTROL OF INDOLEAMINE METABOLISM IN THE RAT PINEAL GLAND

Harry J. Lynch, Maria Hsuan and Richard J. Wurtman

Laboratory of Neuroendocrine Regulation
Department of Nutrition and Food Science
Massachusetts Institute of Technology
Cambridge, Massachusetts 02139

INTRODUCTION

The rate of melatonin biosynthesis in the mammalian pineal gland varies rhythmically. Melatonin secreted from the pineal acts on the brain to modify its biochemical composition (Anton-Tay, 1971) and influence such diverse behavioral and physiological functions as rhythmic locomotor activity patterns (Quay, 1970), the electroencephalogram (Roldan and Anton-Tay, 1968), sleep (Marczynski, Yamaguchi, Ling, and Grodzinska, 1964), and, through its apparent effects on the anterior pituitary, gonadal function and other peripheral endocrine effects (Reiter and Fraschini, 1969). The endocrine rhythms associated with pineal gland function are described by Russel Reiter elsewhere in this volume.

The rhythmic secretion of melatonin from the pineal is thought to impart adaptive advantage to animals by temporally harmonizing cyclic behavioral and physiological processes with daily and seasonal environmental changes. Not surprisingly, the same extraterrestrial input (radiant energy from the sun) that is primarily responsible for cyclically altering the animal's environment also modulates the rate of melatonin biosynthesis in the pineal. The physiological mechanisms underlying this mode of control have been exhaustively explored (Wurtman, Axelrod, and Kelly, 1968). Pineal weight, composition, and biosynthetic activity are temporally cyclic; these cycles have been shown to bear a fixed phase relationship to rhythmic changes in environmental illumination. The first observation suggesting an indirect influence of light on the pineal was reported by Fiske and her collaborators (1960). These investigators' primary interest was to study the mechanism whereby pro-

---

These studies were supported in part by a grant from the United States Public Health Service (AM-11709), and by a grant from the National Aeronautics and Space Administration (NGR-22-009-627). Dr. Lynch holds an NIH Postdoctoral Fellowship (AM-52331-01).

tracted exposure of rats to continuous illumination accelerates their gonadal maturation. They found that a concurrent effect of continuous exposure to environmental illumination for several weeks was a decrease in the weight of the pineal organ. It was then shown that either pinealectomy or exposure to continuous illumination caused equal, non-additive increases in rat gonad weight and that the administration of bovine pineal extracts (Wurtman, Roth, Altschule, and Wurtman, 1961) or the administration of pure solutions of melatonin (Wurtman, Axelrod, and Chu, 1963) blocks the effects of light.

Bioanalytical studies have demonstrated light dependent rhythmic variations in numerous aspects of the composition of the pineal. These include catecholamine content (Wurtman, Axelrod, Sedvall, and Moore, 1967), serotonin and melatonin content (Quay, 1963), and N-acetylserotonin content (Brownstein, Saavedra, and Axelrod, 1973). Similarly, the level of activity of certain pineal enzymes has been found to vary as a function of environmental illumination, e.g., hydroxyindole-O-methyltransferase (Wurtman, Axelrod, and Philips, 1963), L-aromatic amino acid decarboxylase (Snyder, Axelrod, Wurtman, and Fischer, 1965) and serotonin-N-acetyltransferase (Klein and Weller, 1970).

The pathway by which photic control is exerted on the pineal has been and remains the subject of intense study. Meticulous anatomical studies on the rat pineal by Ariens-Kappers (1960) and later on the cat and rabbit pineals by Owman (1965) established that nerve fibers from the superior cervical ganglia provide the major, and perhaps exclusive, sympathetic innervation to the pineal.

Moore and his associates (1967) utilized the phenomenon of light-dependent variations in pineal enzyme activity as a "function test" to identify the brain tracts that mediate the effects of light on pineal biochemical activity. The effects of exposure to continuous light or darkness on pineal hydroxyindole-O-methyltransferase activity were measured in rats previously subjected to lesions of various retinal projections. The neural pathway so revealed includes the following anatomical components: retina, inferior accessory optic tract, medial forebrain bundle, medial terminal nucleus of the accessory optic system, preganlionic sympathetic elements in the spinal cord, superior cervical ganglia, and finally, postganglionic sympathetic fibers (nervi conarii) that terminate near the parenchymal cells of the pineal.

It was subsequently demonstrated (Taylor and Wilson, 1970) that photic stimulation of the rat retina results in a depression in electrical activity in the pineal; whereas, there is a high level of spontaneous electrical activity in the pineal in darkness. This fact accords with the observation that exposure of rats to light lowers catecholamine conent of the pineal (Wurtman, Axelrod, Sedvall and Moore, 1967) and that, as noted above, morphology, biochemical composition, and biosynthetic activity of the pineal have been observed to wax and wane as a function of changes in environmental illumination.

Details of the ultimate link in the chain of neural control of pineal function, i.e., that between the discharge of the postganglionic sympathetic nerve's transmitter substance, norepinephrine, and its biochemical consequences in the pineal parenchymal cell, have been largely illuminated through studies utilizing pineal organ culture techniques

(Shein, Wurtman, and Axelrod, 1967; Shein and Wurtman, 1969; Axelrod, Shein, and Wurtman, 1969; Klein and Rowe, 1969; Klein and Weller, 1970). The mechanism appears to involve stimulation by norepinephrine of a beta-adrenergic receptor on the pinealocyte and subsequent activation of adenylate cyclase which enhances the formation of adenosine 3',5'-cyclic monophosphate (cyclic AMP).

Although environmental lighting constitutes the major factor controlling pineal sympathetic tone and indole biosynthesis, it apparently is not the only factor, inasmuch as significant daily rhythms in hydroxyindole-O-methyltransferase (Nagle, Cardinali, and Rosner, 1972) and N-acetyltransferase (Klein and Weller, 1970) activities and melatonin content (Ralph, Mull, Lynch, and Hedlund, 1971) persist in the pineals of blinded rats and animals maintained under constant darkness.

Recent studies in this laboratory on the effects of adrenergic drugs on pineal biosynthetic activity led to an intriguing incidental observation, namely, that while the subcutaneous injection of L-dopa in saline suspension resulted in a marked increase in pineal melatonin content, he administration of physiological saline alone also elicited a slight increase in pineal melatonin content (Figure 1).

A series of studies was initiated to test the possibility that: 1) sympathetic nervous stimulation, induced by factors other than changes in environmental illumination, might stimulate melatonin biosynthesis in the pineal, and 2) pineal function might be influenced independently of its direct sympathetic input. To this end, rats were subjected to experimentally imposed stress, either insulin induced hypoglycemia or physical immobilization. In view of the observation that prior denervation of the rat pineal resulted in supersensitivity of that organ to L-dopa and exogenous catecholamines (Deguchi and Axelrod, 1972a), the sympathetic neurons of some of the animals in our study were damaged by pretreatment with 6-hydroxydopamine. Either stress modality did stimulate pineal biosynthetic activity in intact animals as evidenced by increases in pineal N-acetyltransferase (NAT) activity and melatonin content, and the response in each case was potentiated by 6-hydroxydopamine pretreatment (Lynch, Eng, and Wurtman, 1973).

The present series of studies was undertaken to further investigate these phenomena using animals whose pineals were surgically denervated. Some animals were adrenalectomized to eliminate one potential source of circulating catecholamines. Animals were subjected to either the systemic stress modalities mentioned above or to alterations in environmental illumination to see if two mechanisms of pineal control could be resolved.

MATERIALS AND METHODS

Intact, adrenalectomized, and superior cervical ganglionectomized male Sprague-Dawley rats weighing 160-200 grams were obtained from the Zivic-Miller Laboratories, Inc., Allison Park, Pennsylvania. Unless otherwise indicated, all rats were maintained under diurnal lighting conditions (lights on from 9 a.m. to 9 p.m.). Illumination, measuring 300 $\mu W/cm^2$, was supplied by "Vita-Lite" fluorescent tubes (Duro-Test Manufacturing Co., North Bergen, N.J.). Big Red Laboratory Animal Diet

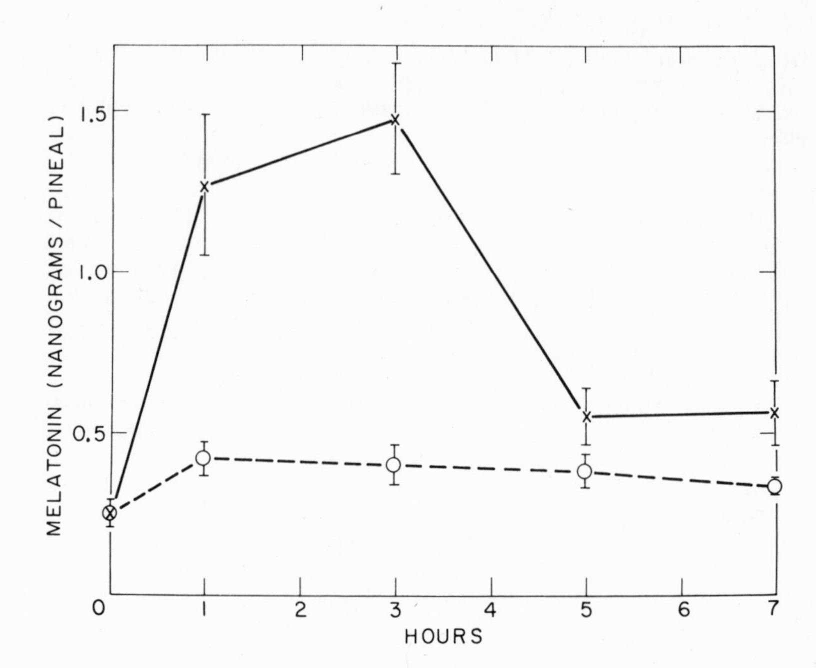

Figure 1. Time-course of pineal melatonin response to L-dopa. Vertical bars indicate standard errors of the mean. The solid line represents pineal melatonin content of rats killed at intervals after subcutaneous injection of L-dopa (300 mg/kg of body weight) in saline suspension. The dotted line represents pineal melatonin content of rats receiving only the vehicle. Figure from Lynch, Wang, and Wurtman, 1973.

and water were available ad libitum. All adrenalectomized animals were given drinking water containing 1% NaCl. Those that were treated with 6-hydroxydopamine (6-OHDA) and/or subjected to physical immobilization were injected subcutaneously with 1 mg of corticosterone in sesame oil daily prior to the experiment.

Some animals were subjected to a partial chemical sympathectomy, accomplished through a series of intravenous (tail vein) injections of 6-hydroxydopamine (Thoenen and Tranzer, 1968). Each animal treated received two injections (34 mg/kg each in 0.001 N HCl) 12 days before the experiment and two additional injections (68 mg/kg each) one week later.

All experiments involving physical immobilization were performed between 10 a.m. and 2 p.m. Immobilization was accomplished by securing each animal to a fiberboard stock with adhesive tape; control animals remained undisturbed in their cages. After 2 hours, all of the animals were killed by decapitation and their pineal glands quickly removed. Pineals to be assayed for melatonin content were frozen in 1.0 ml of deionized water and bioassayed within 3 days. Pineals to be assayed for N-acetyltransferase (NAT) activity were initially frozen on dry ice and assayed within 14 hours. Pineal melatonin content was estimated by a quantitative bioassay based on the response of dermal melanophores in larval anurans to melatonin present in their bathing medium (Ralph and Lynch, 1970). Light-adapted Rana pipiens larvae were placed in dilute pineal homogenates. The melatonin content was then estimated by comparing the extent of nucleocentric melanin aggregation that resulted in the dermal melanophores of these animals with that observed in tadpoles similarly exposed to known concentrations of authentic melatonin. Pineal N-acetyltransferase activity was determined by a modification of the method of Deguchi and Axelrod (1972b) which involves measuring the transfer of a ^{14}C-acetyl moiety from acetyl coenzyme A to tryptamine. Each pineal was homogenized in a mixture containing 3.5 μmole of potassium phosphate (pH 6.5) and 0.17 μmole of tryptamine. Two nmole of ^{14}C-acetyl coenzyme A (New England Nuclear, Boston, Mass.; specific activity 49.8 mCi/mmole) were added to yield a final volume of 70 μl. After incubation at 37°C for 15 min, the reaction was stopped by the addition of 1.0 ml of 0.5 M borate buffer (pH 10) and the ^{14}C-N-acetyltryptamine was extracted into 6 ml of a mixture of toluene and iso-amyl alcohol (97:3). After centrifugation, 4 ml of the organic phase was transferred to a scintillation vial and evaporated. The residue was dissolved in 1 ml of absolute ethanol; 10 ml of toluene-based phosphor was added, and the radioactivity was measured in a liquid scintillation spectrometer.

RESULTS

1. Effects of Physical Immobilization on Pineal Biosynthetic Activity Following Various Surgical and Pharmacological Treatments

Pineal N-acetyltransferase (NAT) activity (Klein and Weller, 1970) and melatonin content (Quay, 1963; Lynch, 1971) are lowest during the light phase among rats exposed to a diurnal lighting schedule. Intact animals stressed for 2 hours, by being immobilized, and kept in the light during this interval exhibit significant increases in pineal NAT activity and melatonin content. These effects are markedly potentiated by pretreatment with systemic 6-hydroxydopamine (Lynch, Eng, and Wurtman, 1973). Prior surgical denervation of the pineal by bilateral superior cervical ganglionectomy similarly potentiates both of its responses to immobilization (Figure 2, Table 1). Animals previously subjected to bilateral adrenalectomy fail to display increases in pineal NAT following physical immobilization; however, if they have also been subjected

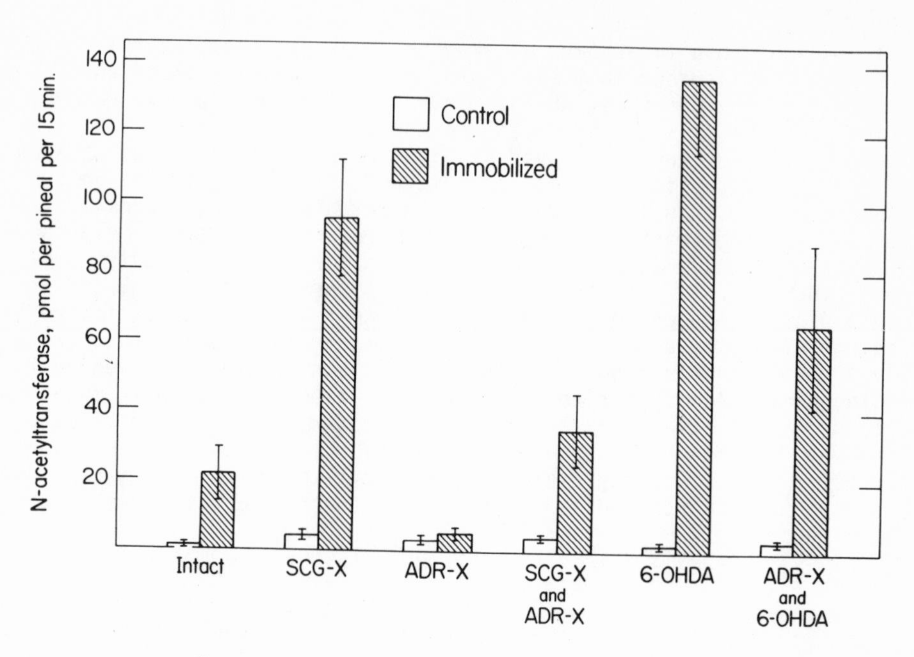

Figure 2. Effect of physical immobilization on rat pineal N-acetyltransferase activity following superior cervical ganglionectomy (SCG-X), adrenalectomy (ADR-X) and/or 6-hydroxydopamine (6-OHDA) treatment. Groups of 4-9 rats were rendered immobile by being secured individually to fiberboard stocks with adhesive tape. They were killed 2 hours later. Control animals remained undisturbed in their cages and were killed at the same time as the corresponding experimental group. Vertical lines indicate standard error of the mean.

to ganglionectomy or pretreated with 6-hydroxydopamine, pineal NAT does respond to immobilization (Figure 2). Pineal melatonin content does not increase in immobilized rats that have been subjected to both adrenalectomy and ganglionectomy (Table 1). The mechanism of this dissociation between NAT activity and melatonin content is now known; however, the phenomenon suggests that NAT activity is not always the major factor controlling melatonin synthesis.

Pretreatment with the alpha-adrenergic blocking agent, phenoxybenzamine, increases pineal NAT activity as reported by Deguchi and Axelrod (1972a), potentiates the pineal NAT response to physical immobilization in intact animals (Figure 3), and restores the NAT response to immobilization in adrenalectomized rats (Figure 3).

TABLE 1. EFFECT OF PHYSICAL IMMOBILIZATION ON PINEAL MELATONIN CONTENT FOLLOWING SURGICAL DENERVATION OF THE PINEAL OR DENERVATION AND ADRENALECTOMY.

	Pineal melatonin content ng/pineal			
Surgical preparation	Control		Immobilized	
None	(5)	0.10 ± 0.06	(5)	1.09 ± 0.24[a]
Ganglionectomy	(5)	0.21 ± 0.05	(4)	1.89 ± 0.39[a,b]
Ganglionectomy + Adrenalectomy	(5)	0.21 ± 0.02	(4)	0.20 ± 0.10[c]

Groups of intact and surgically prepared animals were rendered immobile by being secured individually to fiberboard stocks and were killed 2 hours later. Control animals remained undisturbed in their cages.
The results are expressed as mean ± standard error of the mean. The figure in parenthesis indicates the number of animals in that experimental group.

[a] *$P < 0.005$ differs from corresponding control animals.*

[b] *$P < 0.005$ differs from intact immobilized animals.*

[c] *Not significantly different from corresponding control animals.*

2. Effects of Changes in Environmental Illumination on Pineal Biosynthetic Activity Following Various Surgical and Pharmacological Treatments

Untreated rats exposed to a diurnal lighting schedule exhibit a 15- to 40-fold daily variation in the level of pineal NAT activity (Klein and Weller, 1970). The amplitude of this daily variation is increased in rats pretreated with systemic 6-hydroxydopamine, and the anticipated rise in NAT activity after the onset of darkness is abolished by ganglionectomy (Figure 4). The nocturnal rise is not restored in ganglionecomized rats by pretreatment with 6-hydroxydopamine (Figure 4).

After protracted exposure to continuous illumination (10 days), the magnitude of the increase in pineal NAT activity after 3 hours of darkness is several fold greater than that observed in animals experiencing daily photoperiods (Figure 5). Adrenalectomy, which blocks pineal response to immobilization (Figure 2), does not block the increase in NAT activity occurring when rats are placed in darkness (Figure 5).

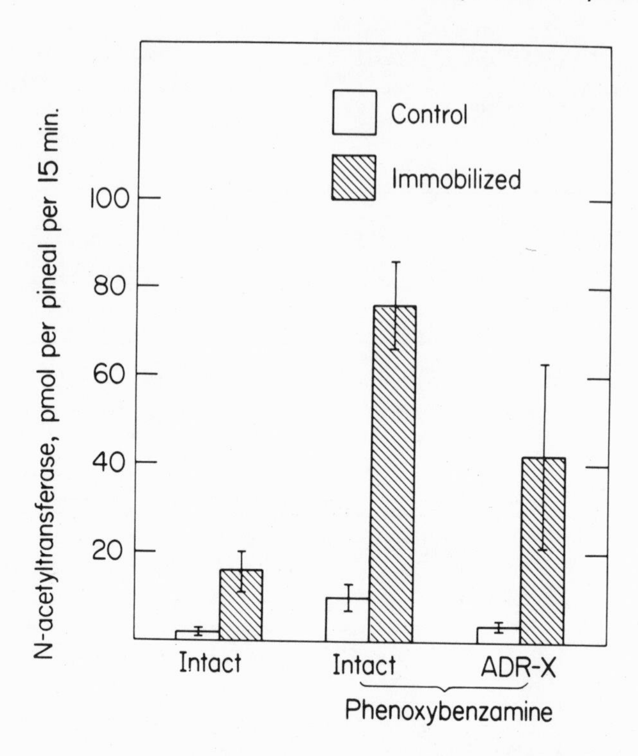

Figure 3. Effect of physical immobilization on pineal N-acetyltransferase activity in intact and adrenalectomized rats following pretreatment with phenoxybenzamine. Groups of 7 rats were maintained under constant light for 72 hours. Phenoxybenzamine (20 mg/kg body weight) in 0.5 ml saline solution was injected subcutaneously to all rats 30 minutes before subgroups were immobilized for two hours. Vertical lines indicate standard error of the mean.

DISCUSSION

The mechanisms underlying the acceleration in rat pineal biosynthetic activity brought about by either rendering the animals immobile or by exposing them to darkness appear to differ. The response to immobilization can be effectively abolished by adrenalectomy but not by the surgical or chemical denervation of the pineal, i.e., with 6-hydroxydopamine (Figure 2). In contrast, superior cervical ganglionectomy blocks the pineal response to darkness; while adrenalectomy has no effect on this phenomenon (Figure 5). These observations suggest that pineal

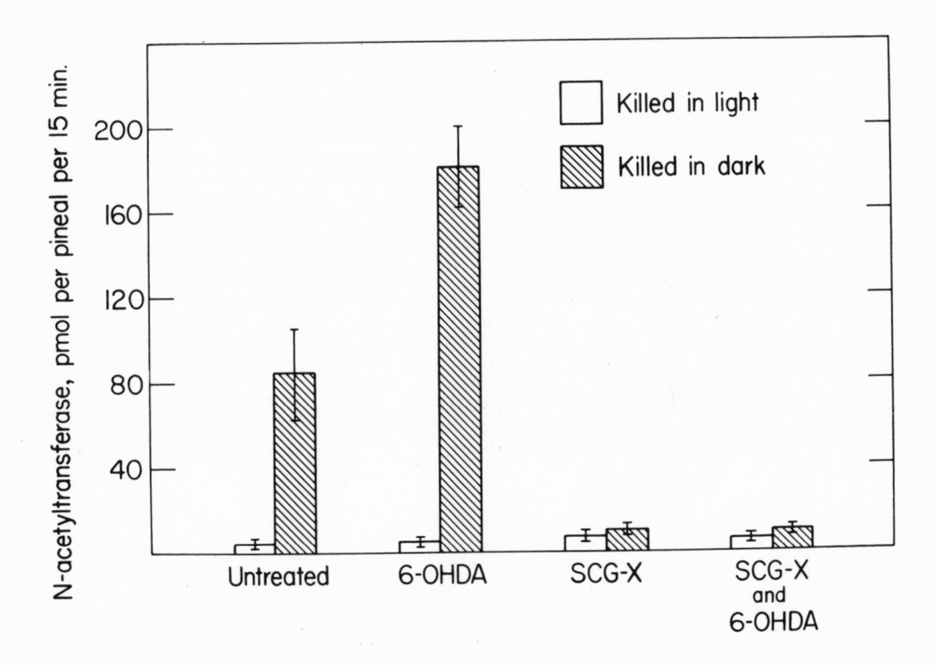

Figure 4. Effect of environmental illumination on pineal N-acetyltransferase activity following various surgical and/or pharmacological treatments: Groups of 5 or 6 rats were maintained under a diurnal lighting schedule with lights on from 9 a.m. to 9 p.m. Subgroups were killed either at 12:00 midnight, 3 hours after the onset of darkness, or at 12:00 noon, 3 hours after the onset of light. Vertical lines indicate standard error of the mean.

NAT activity can be enhanced either by the release of norepinephrine from sympathetic terminals within the pineal or by circulating catecholamines liberated from the adrenal medulla and from sympathetic nerve terminals elsewhwere in the body. The stress of immobilization, by increasing circulating catecholamines, stimulates the pineal; the onset of darkness apparently does not cause a sufficient rise in circulating catecholamines to do so, and thus the photic control of pineal function requires intact pineal sympathetic innervation.

Using histochemical fluorescence as a criterion, Eränkö and Eränkö (1971) failed to detect catecholamines in the pineals of rats treated neonatally with 6-hydroxydopamine; similarly, we found no chemically-assayable norepinephrine in pooled pineals of 10 adult rats treated as

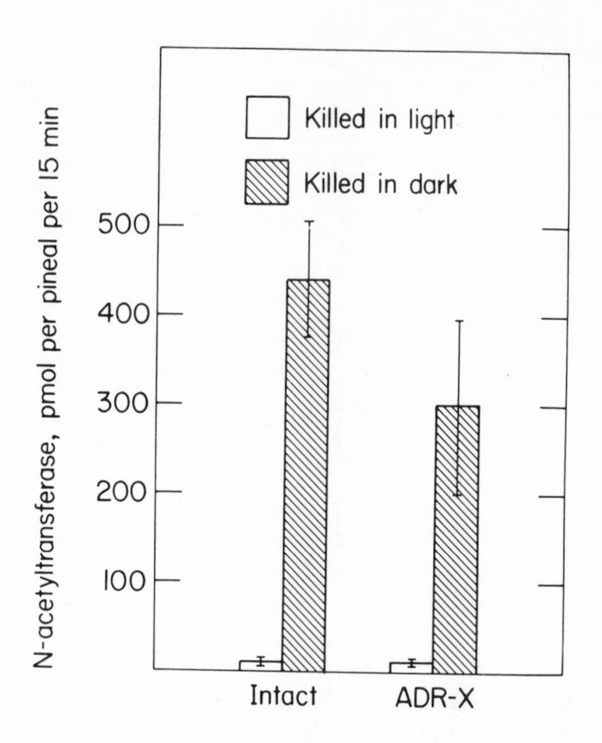

Figure 5. Effect of environmental illumination on pineal N-acetyltransferase activity following adrenalectomy. Groups of 6 or 7 rats were maintained in constant light for 10 days. Subgroups were then placed in total darkness for 3 hours. Vertical lines indicate standard error of the mean.

described above with 6-hydroxydopamine. Just the same, we suspect that total sympathetic denervation was not attained in our animals treated with 6-hydroxydopamine. That such treatment potentiates the pineal NAT response to darkness, which requires pineal sympathetic innervation, and that ganglionectomy or pretreatment with 6-hydroxydopamine in combination with ganglionectomy completely abolishes this response (Figure 4) suggest that the 6-hydroxydopamine treatment alone, while rendering the pineal supersensitive to adrenergic stimulation, does not totally eliminate its sympathetic input.

The mediation by beta-adrenergic receptors of the effects of norepinephrine on pineal biosynthetic activity is well known (Wurtman, Shein, and Larin, 1971) and the blockade of the pineal NAT response to physical immobilization by propranolol, a beta-adrenergic blocking agent, has been demonstrated (Lynch, Eng, and Wurtman, 1973). The stimulation of pineal NAT in vivo by the alpha-adrenergic blocking agent, phenoxybenzamine, has been reported by Deguchi and Axelrod (1972a) and is confirmed in the studies reported here (Figure 3). Klein and Weller (1973) report a similar effect in vitro of the alpha-adrenergic blocking agent, phentolamine. Just how beta-adrenergic stimulation can be influenced by alpha-adrenergic blockade remains to be explained. The in vivo observations reported here may help to extend the utility of the pineal gland as a model for biochemical and pharmacological studies of neural control of end organs, adrenergic receptor sites and the resolution of diverse physiological functions that are under sympathetic control.

The adaptive significance of the alternative modes of control of the pineal that these studies suggest remains to be elucidated. The relative contributions of each to the net secretory activity of the pineal may vary from one mammalian species to another and may correlate with the ecological niches occupied by various animals. For example, it is possible that among animals living in the earth's temperate zones, where there are marked annual variations in the length of the daily hotoperiod, the pineal serves to synchronize cyclic reproductive funcions with seasonal variables. In the tropics, where marked rhythmic changes in the length of photoperiod do not occur, other environmental variables may, by influencing sympathetic tone or plasma catecholamine concentrations, control pineal function.

Melatonin secretion from the pineal may have physiologic consequences not hitherto considered. If, as the present studies suggest, non-specific stress triggers increased biosynthesis and secretion of melatonin, this hormone may participate in mechanisms of adaptation that remain to be characterized.

REFERENCES

Anton-Tay, F. (1971). Pineal brain relationships. In: *The Pineal Gland* (Wolstenholm, G. E. W. and Knight, J., eds.), pp. 213-227, Churchill Livingston, London.

Ariens-Kappers, J. (1960). Innervation of the epiphysis cerebri in the albino rat. Anat. Rec. 136, 220-227.

Axelrod, J., Shein, H., and Wurtman, R. J. (1969). Stimulation of ^{14}C-melatonin synthesis from ^{14}C-tryptophan by noradrenalin in rat pineal organ culture. Proc. Natl. Acad. Sci., U.S.A. 62, 544-549.

Brownstein, M., Saavedra, J. M., and Axelrod, J. (1973). Control of pineal N-acetylserotonin by a beta-adrenergic receptor. Mol. Pharmacol. 9, 605-611.

Deguchi, T. and Axelrod, J. (1972a). Induction and superinduction of serotonin N-acetyltransferase by adrenergic drugs and denervation in rat pineal organ. Proc. Nat. Acad. Sci., U.S.A. 69, 2208-2211.

Deguchi, T. and Axelrod, J. (1972b). Sensitive assay for serotonin-N-acetyltransferase activity in rat pineal. Anal. Biochem. 50, 174-179.

Eränkö, O. and Eränkö, L. (1971). Loss of histochemically demonstrable catecholamines and acetylcholinesterase from sympathetic nerve fibers of the pineal body of the rat after chemical sympathectomy with 6-hydroxydopamine. Histochem. J. 3, 357-363.

Fiske, V. M., Bryant, K., and Putnam, J. (1960). Effect of light on weight of the pineal in the rat. Endocrinology 66, 489-491.

Klein, D. C. and Weller, J. L. (1970). Indole metabolism in the pineal gland: a circadian rhythm in N-acetyltransferase. Science 169, 1093-1095.

Klein, D. C. and Weller, J. L. (1973). Adrenergic-adenosine 3'5'-monophosphate regulation of serotonin N-acetyltransferase activity and the temporal relationship of serotonin N-acetyltransferase activity to the synthesis of ^{3}H-N-acetylserotonin and ^{3}H-melatonin in the cultured rat pineal gland. J. Pharmacol. Exp. Therap. 186, 516-527.

Lynch, H. J. (1971). Diurnal oscillations in pineal melatonin content. Life Sci. 10, 791-795.

Lynch, H. J., Eng, J. P., and Wurtman, R. J. (1973). Control of pineal indole biosynthesis by changes in sympathetic tone caused by factors other than environmental lighting. Proc. Natl. Acad. Sci., U.S.A. 70, 1704-1707.

Lynch, H. J., Wang, P., and Wurtman, R. J. (1973). Increase in rat pineal melatonin content following L-dopa administration. Life Sci. 12, 145-151.

Marczynski, T. J., Yamaguchi, N., Ling, G. M., and Grodzinska, L. (1964). Sleep induced by the administration of melatonin (5-methoxy-N-acetyl-tryptamine) to the hypothalamus of unrestrained cats. Experientia 20, 435-437.

Moore, R. Y., Heller, A., Wurtman, R. J., and Axelrod, J. (1967). Visual pathways mediating pineal response to environmental lighting. Science 155, 220-223.

Nagle, C. A., Cardinali, D. P., and Rosner, J. M. (1972). Light regulation of rat retinal hydroxyindole-O-methyltransferase (HIOMT) activity. Endocrinology 91, 423-426.

Owman, C. (1965). Localization of neural and parenchymal monamines under normal and experimental conditions in the mammalian pineal gland. Prog. Brain Res. 10, 423-453.

Quay, W. B. (1970). Precocious entrainment and associated characteristics of activity patterns following pinealectomy and reversal of photoperiod. Physiol. Behav. 5, 1281-1290.

Quay, W. B. (1963). Circadian rhythm in rat pineal serotonin and its modifications by estrous cycle and photoperiod. Gen. Comp. Endocrinol. 3, 473-479.

Ralph, C. L. and Lynch, H. J. (1970). A quantitative melatonin bioassay. Gen. Comp. Endocrinol. 15, 334-338.

Ralph, C. L., Mull, D., Lynch, H. J., and Hedlund, L. (1971). A melatonin rhythm persists in rat pineals in darkness. Endocrinology 89, 1361-1366.

Reiter, R. J. and Fraschini, F. (1969). Endocrine aspects of the mammalian pineal gland: a review. Neuroendocrinology 5, 219-255.

Roldan, E. and Anton-Tay, F. (1968). EEG and convulsive threshold changes produced by pineal extract administration. Brain Res. 11, 238-245.

Snyder, S. H., Axelrod, J., Wurtman, R. J. and Fischer, J. E. (1965). Control of 5-hydroxytryptophan decarboxylase activity in the rat pineal gland by sympathetic nerves. J. Pharmacol. Exp. Therap. 147, 371-375.

Shein, H., Wurtman, R. J., and Axelrod, J. (1967). Serotonin synthesis in pineal gland in organ culture. Nature 213, 730-731.

Shein, H. M. and Wurtman, R. J. (1969). Cyclic adenosine monophosphate: stimulation of melatonin and serotonin synthesis in cultured rat pineals. Science 166, 519-520.

Taylor, A. N. and Wilson, R. W. (1970). Electrophysiological evidence for the action of light on the pineal gland in the rat. Experientia 26, 267-269.

Thoenen, H. and Tranzer, J. P. (1968). Chemical sympathectomy by selective destruction of adrenergic nerve endings with 6-hydroxydopamine. Arch. Exp. Pathol. Pharmacol. 261, 271-288.

Wurtman, R. J., Altschule, M. D., and Holmgren, U. (1959). Effects of pinealectomy and of a bovine pineal extract on rats. Am. J. Physiol. 197, 108-110.

Wurtman, R. J., Axelrod, J., and Chu, E. W. (1963). Melatonin, a pineal substance: its effect on the rat ovary. Science 141, 277-278.

Wurtman, R. J., Axelrod, J., and Fischer, J. E. (1964). Melatonin synthesis in the pineal gland: effect of light mediated by the sympathetic nervous system. Science 143, 1328-1330.

Wurtman, R. J., Axelrod, J. and Kelly, D. E. (1968). *The Pineal.* Academic Press, New York.

Wurtman, R. J., Axelrod, J. and Phillips, L. (1963). Melatonin synthesis in the pineal gland: control by light. Science 142, 1071-1073.

Wurtman, R. J., Axelrod, J., Sedvall, G. and Moore, R. Y. (1967). Photic and neural control of the 24-hour norepinephrine rhythm in the rat pineal gland. J. Pharmacol. Exptl. Therap. 157, 487-492.

Wurtman, R. J., Roth, W., Altschule, M. D., and Wurtman, J. J. (1961). Interactions of the pineal and exposure to continuous light on organ weights of female rats. Acta. Endocrinol. 36, 617-624.

Wurtman, R. J., Shein, H. M. and Larin, F. (1971). Mediation by β-adrenergic receptors of effect of norepinephrine on pineal synthesis of ^{14}C-serotonin and ^{14}C-melatonin. J. Neurochem. 18, 1683-1687.

DISCUSSION AFTER DR. LYNCH'S PAPER

Dr. Reiter

Undoubtedly, there are species which inhabit the Tropics that are continuous breeders and there are others which inhabit the Tropics that are seasonal breeders. Also, your point about other things cueing pineal activity is very well taken. There are some circannual cycles, for example, that are synchronized by rainfall and some synchronized by other environmental factors such as ambient temperature. These changes may have something to do with determining pineal activity. There are other species that you can move from the Temperate Zone, such as the Sika deer, which is normally a seasonal breeder, into the Tropics and it becomes a continuous breeder. This would be anticipated because the pineal gland probably has a great deal to do with determining seasonal reproductive phenomena. When a temperate species is moved to a tropical or subtropical area where the photoperiod is relatively constant throughout the year, the animal may become capable of continuous reproduction.

I have a couple of questions. I still don't quite understand the slide where you gave 6-hydroxydopamine and you said, on the basis of your results, that probably 6-hydroxydopamine failed to cause degeneration of the noradrenergic terminals (see Figure 4). If that is true, as best I could tell, the response was in fact potentiated in the darkness in these animals. How do you explain this?

Dr. Lynch

Indeed, the pineal NAT response to darkness was potentiated by pretreatment with 6-hydroxydopamine (6-OHDA), and it is for this reason that I suspect sympathetic denervation of the pineal was not complete. Figure 4 also showed that bilateral superior cervical ganglionectomy, either alone or in combination with 6-OHDA treatment, abolished the response to darkness. Although we were unable to detect norepinephrine fluorometrically in the pooled pineals of ten rats following the 6-OHDA treatment, enough of the sympathetic input evidently remained intact to mediate the pineal response to environmental lighting changes. Here, I think, partial chemical sympathectomy rendered the pineal super-sensitive to adrenergic stimulation. So, despite the diminished input, the pineal NAT response was potentiated.

Dr. Reiter

Pharmacological and histochemical evidence indicates the pineal apparently also has a cholinergic innervation. Have you ever tested the effect of acetylcholine on any of the enzymes within the pineal gland and have you gotten any effect? Secondly, have you tested the ubiquitously acting prostaglandins as to their potential role in regulating the synthesis of the pineal indoles?

Dr. Lynch

No, we have not made an effort to investigate the involvement of either acetylcholine or prostaglandins in the regulation of pineal function.

Dr. Ramaley

I'm interested in the role of circulating catecholamines which you were trying to illustrate here. I gather, in general, that in the basal state of the normal diurnal rhythm rate you do not feel they probably affect the pineal because if you remove the adrenal, you don't see a change in your enzyme activity. Is that right?

Dr. Lynch

That is right.

Dr. Ramaley

In the stress state, however, you feel that the discharge from the adrenal is important. What is the normal diurnal rhythm in the rat? Is it the same as in the human, that is, high levels during the day; or is it the reciprocal of the human? I'm still interested in the question of the relationship between pineal rhythms and blood catecholamine rhythms in the rat. Are they high during the day or during the night? Secondly, if you remove the adrenal entirely, does the rhythm disappear? That is, is the adrenal the main source of this rhythm or are there effects of peripheral catecholamine secretion?

Dr. Lynch

I do not know if there is a normal cyclic change in the concentration of catecholamines in rat blood. If there is, it is simply unmeasurable with the analytical methods we have at our disposal now.

However, I do believe that these and earlier studies (Deguchi and Axelrod, 1972; Lynch et al., 1973) amply demonstrate that the NAT response of the denervated pineal is an exquisitely sensitive indicator of circulating catecholamines. Because the pineals of ganglionectomized rats do not respond to the transition from environmental lighting to darkness, I conclude that if there is an increase in the concentration of blood-borne catecholamines with the onset of darkness, it is very meager.

As for the relative contributions of the adrenals and peripheral catecholamine secretion in mediating the pineal NAT response to stress, I think the fact that surgically denervated pineals of adrenalectomized rats respond to physical immobilization suggests that NAT activity can be enhanced by norepinephrine released from sympathetic nerve terminals elsewhere in the body.

Dr. Reiter

I'm becoming a little concerned about what exactly the role of light is in determining melatonin synthesis. The rhythms of melatonin, HIOMT, and N-acetyltransferase persist in constant dark-exposed or blinded animals. Wouldn't it be just as logical to assume that what really happens is that as melatonin is synthesized in darkness, it accumulates within the pineal gland and feeds back to inhibit its own synthesis? This would explain the ostensible diurnal rhythm in animals kept in alternating photoperiods and would also explain the rhythm which persists in dark-exposed animals.

Dr. Lynch

That is certainly a consideration. In the paper cited earlier, Weiss (1968) presents data showing that the addition of melatonin to incubation mixtures does indeed inhibit HIOMT activity in vitro. Whether endogenously formed melatonin exerts a physiological control over its own synthesis remains to be established. This may be rather difficult. Here we have seen that on immobilization of adrenalectomized rats there is a dramatic increase in NAT activity in denervated pineals while there is no increase in pineal melatonin content. Elsewhere, we have shown that when animals were pre-treated with the beta-adrenergic blocking agent, propranolol, the increase in NAT activity on immobilization was substantially blocked while pineal melatonin content was increased (Lynch et al., 1973). Both of these phenomena may reflect an alteration in the rate of melatonin secretion from the pineal that is attributable to cardiovascular changes induced by the treatments.

Dr. Krieger

I was just wondering about the effect of the adrenalectomy which is so interesting. Can you separate the effect of catecholaminergic influences as seen in the stress response and those of adrenal cortical secretion also seen in stress? In other words, you're removing both when you're doing the adrenalectomy.

Dr. Lynch

In those studies involving experimentally imposed stress, our adrenalectomized rats were maintained on a milligram of corticosterone per rat daily. Where we merely sought to test the pineal NAT response to darkness, corticosterone was not administered and the operated animals were maintained on 1% NaCl in their drinking water.

Dr. Krieger

With the constant daily dose of corticosterone you're still not getting the increment of adrenal corticosteroids that you would get in a stress situation. In other words, what's happening during stress in an adrenalectomized animal maintained on corticosterone is that you're allowing for the permissive action of corticosterone but you're not allowing for a stress increment. It might be a change in gradient of steroid levels to which the pineal is responding.

Dr. Lynch

Yes, you may be right.

Dr. Kitay

I wonder if you could comment a bit further about the point you made a moment ago about the lack of information concerning melatonin secretion. One of your points was that there was a lack of correlation between pineal N-acetyltransferase activity on the one hand and melatonin content in the pineal on the other. You apparently have evidence going both ways for the two parameters. Are there data which in any way relate pineal melatonin content or the activity of any of the enzymes concerned with melatonin synthesis with direct measurement of melatonin secretion or evidence of its peripheral activity? Are there data that might suggest a lack of correlation of pineal melatonin content with evidence of activity?

Dr. Lynch

A possible peripheral manifestation of pineal function is its influence on rhythmic spontaneous locomotor activity in animals. This is the only area in which we have looked for a correlation between pineal function as evidenced by cyclic oscillations in melatonin content and peripheral effects. We wanted to explore the possibility that variations in pineal biosynthetic activity continued to cycle rhythmically under constant environmental conditions. There had been reports suggesting that pineal melatonin biosynthesis ceases to oscillate under conditions of constant light or constant darkness. Such a conclusion might result from sampling at inappropriate times. So, rather than kill groups of animals at arbitrary "clock intervals," we used an experimental approach suggested by Dr. Hedlund.

To demonstrate the persistent oscillation in rat pineal serotonin content in constant darkness, Dr. Hedlund used the ingenious ploy of monitoring the animal's individual locomotor activity pattern and sampling with reference to the phase, i.e., the active or quiescent period of this free-running circadian cyclic behavior.

When we applied this technique and measured pineal melatonin content, we found that in rats in constant darkness melatonin content was high during the active period and low during the quiescent period. Under diurnal lighting conditions, of course, rats are active in the dark and inactive in the light. When chickens in constant darkness were similarly studied, we found melatonin content high during the inactive period and low during the active period, which for chickens under diurnal lighting would correspond to the dark and light phases, respectively.

Though no causal relationship can be inferred from these observations, it is clear that the daily variation in pineal melatonin content and spontaneous locomotor activity are free-running, phase-locked phenomena and that one can be used to predict the phase of the other.

Dr. Reiter

I think the fact that the rhythms persist in the light deprived animal is very interesting and brings up a critical point relative to the role of melatonin. The best I can understand from what I saw in your presentation is that there is the same total amount of melatonin synthesized in the animal exposed to alternating photoperiods as in the animal that is exposed to continuous darkness. And yet we know that continuous darkness has a greater antigonadotrophic effect than alternating photoperiods. This being so, we have to assume one of two things. Either melatonin secretion rate is different in animals exposed to constant darkness than it is in animals exposed to alternating photoperiods, or secondly, the sensitivity of the animal to melatonin is greater in constant darkness than it is in animals kept in alternating photoperiodic conditions. The third possibility is that melatonin is not the pineal antigonadotrophic factor.

Dr. Lynch

Of course, our notion that the rate of melatonin secretion is a direct function of the rate of melatonin biosynthesis rests on the fact that melatonin is a lipid soluble compound and should rapidly escape the cell of origin, no subcellular structure has been demonstrated that might represent a storage particle for melatonin, and the pineal lacks the enzymatic machinery that would be necessary to further metabolize melatonin. Until we are able to measure directly the rate of melatonin secretion from the pineal, I guess we shouldn't rule out the possibility that the process of secretion is under a separate control mechanism.

Dr. Reiter

Has anyone ever looked at the level of melatonin, the activity of HIOMT, serotonin rhythm, or the activity of N-acetyltransferase in animals kept under natural photoperiodic conditions?

Dr. Lynch

You have raised a very important point, Dr. Reiter. I think that your work, elucidating the relationships among the natural photoperiod, the pineal gland, and reproduction in golden hamsters, implicates the pineal in normal mammalian physiology more compellingly than anything else in the literature. The data that we collect on pineal function in the albino rat under experimentally manipulated photoperiodic conditions are certainly contrived. The redeeming value of this work is that it has enabled us to develop methods for the direct assessment of pineal function and to learn something about the nature of its control. We must now apply this technology in the study of animal populations that are subject to natural environmental variables in the field.

Dr. Karsch

I agree that it is essential to look at the role of the pineal in animals maintained in their own natural environment. In this regard, the effect of pinealectomy on the occurrence of breeding seasons is of particular interest. However, if breeding seasons persist for several years in the absence of the pineal, as Dr. Reiter indicated in his presentation, this will be an extremely difficult phenomenon to examine experimentally.

Dr. Reiter

In the experiment on the ferret it wasn't quite a year that the system was programmed; they were pinealectomized in October and came into estrus the following April, roughly a six to seven month period. I think we talked about an experiment during the recess where one could, in fact, test when the programming occurs. If one pinealectomized some animals in October, as Herbert did, some in September, some in August, and subsequently, one could identify when the programming takes place. I think this would be a very interesting experiment.

Dr. Halberg

Were you involved in studies on any relation of pineal function to feeding mechanisms?

Dr. Lynch

No, we have not worked on that phase yet.

Dr. Halberg

We have had some correspondence with Dr. Kolpakov of Novosibirsk on questions studied also by Dean R. Andrews of Creighton University in Nebraska. Both attempted to assess circannual rhythms in vitro. If such were found you would have good proof of endogenous behavior, as considered by Dr. Reiter. To turn back to in vivo data, in addition to the catfish investigation of Professor Sundararaj, Professor Y. Benoit of Paris kept ducks in continuous light for about five years and some other ducks in continuous darkness for quite a while. By inspection of the original data and by curve fitting associated with a zero amplitude test, changes were uncovered that appeared to be non-random. In addition to such behavioral evidence, usually involving more than weights, biochemical in vitro results remain desirable.

With respect to your very fine presentation, you brought home the point forcefully that a major circannual rhythm in human beings, that of urinary norepinephrine and epinephrine, may perhaps interact with the pineal gland and you have provided experimental evidence in support of this point. Is this correct?

Dr. Lynch

Yes, sir, I feel that we have.

Dr. Dellmann

You showed that the pineal content of melatonin is high at four o'clock in the morning and quite low at eight o'clock in the morning (see Reiter, Figure 6, this volume). I'm wondering at exactly what time does the decrease occur, when you turn on the lights? And a second question: Is it a decreased biosynthesis or an increased release which occurs at that moment?

Dr. Lynch

That's exactly the central question. You're right. When we did the time course studies in the rat we saw a high point at 4 A.M., two hours before the lights came on, and we saw a very low point two hours after the lights were on. Whether it started down before dawn, I don't know. But in the case of the chicken it clearly did. The chicken pineal contained a maximum amount of melatonin at twelve midnight; at four A.M. there was significantly less; and then at eight A.M. there was still less. In the case of the rat it appears that the melatonin content of the pineal increases through the dark and drops abruptly with the onset of light.

Dr. Hedlund

I was confused by one of the observations that you made. Treatment of adrenalectomized rats with 6-hydroxydopamine did not appear to prevent the increase in N-acetyltransferase activity upon immobilization. Is that correct?

Dr. Lynch

There was an increase in the pineal NAT activity upon immobilization following adrenalectomy and 6-hydroxydopamine treatment. It was not so marked as the increase following 6-hydroxydopamine treatment in otherwise intact animals. I believe that the reason for that is the fact that treatment with 6-hydroxydopamine had rendered the pineal supersensitive to catecholamines and that treatment with 6-hydroxydopamine does not destroy all potential sources of catecholamines.

Mr. Friend

Does anyone know the frequency of Horner's syndrome and particularly if it occurs bilaterally? It would seem that Horner's syndrome might be a workable human model in relation to the "cutting off" of the pineal gland due to the ablation of the superior cervical ganglion.

Dr. Krieger

Clinically, I think that one would have to have a patient with bilateral cervical ganglionectomy for an effective model. Virtually, any of the causes of Horner's syndrome that I can think of are usually associated with unilateral findings so you would not have the same kind of human model to study as you would in the animal.

Dr. Reiter

Along this line I would just like to say that the Japanese have pinealectomized individuals with pineal tumors, and unfortunately, there has never been, to my knowledge, any follow-up studies on the endocrine status of these individuals. I would be very curious to see if there were any effects of pinealectomy in the human.

Dr. Halberg

One of the things we thought was established for a long time and amenable to generalization was the difference in timing between many circadian rhythms in nocturnal and diurnal animals. Zola Cooper, so many years ago, scheduled circumcisions around the clock, took prepuces from these infants and found that at night there were more mitoses in the foreskin than by day.

In a study on human beings, Professor Larry Scheving of the Medical Center at Little Rock, Arkansas, including the skin of his own back, showed that mitosis of the epidermis undergoes a circadian rhythm with drastic amplitude, a finding confirmed by Fisher in England quite a few years later (Halberg et al., 1973). The mitotic rhythm in human epidermis is about 180° out of phase with that in epidermis of nocturnal rodents. Similar differences have been found by us for rhythms in body core temperature, blood eosinophil counts, serum corticoid, and many more variables.

It is more interesting to see that under natural conditions of light and darkness in the laboratory, melatonin in human blood and in the blood of rodents is in phase in terms of timing of rhythms. That is, during the dark span you have an increase both in rat and in man. Is this correct?

Dr. Lynch
Yes.

Dr. Halberg
Your findings prompt one to consider data with chlorothiazide-induced saluresis, diuresis, and kaliuresis. We have studied these phenomena with Mr. Ronald Shiotsuka of our laboratory and also with Dr. Howard Levine of New Britain, Connecticut, in normotensive and hypertensive rats and healthy hospital resident physicians in New Britain, Connecticut. We developed a chronotherapeutic index (CTI) formed from two ratios. The numerator was the ratio (relative to saline-injected controls) of chlorothiazide-induced saluresis and the denominator an equivalent ratio for potassium. The CTI's indicate the optimal compromise between tending to minimize undesired hypocholemic effects while tending to maximize the desired saluresis. Since there was a similar timing in man and rat, I wonder whether the mechanism may not involve an agent acting upon body rhythms that are also similarly timed in the two species rather than being timed with a difference in acrophase so prominent for many functions other than melatonin. I wonder whether the mechanism may not involve an agent acting upon body rhythms that are also similarly timed in the two species rather than being timed with a difference in acrophase so prominent for many functions other than melatonin. I wonder whether some of you might be interested in checking for a thiazide effect on melatonin.

Dr. Lynch
Dr. Reiter showed an illustration (Reiter, Figure 7, this volume) from Pelham et al. (1973) documenting the diurnal variation in human plasma melatonin content. I've made similar observations on myself by collecting blood at three o'clock in the afternoon and at three o'clock in the morning and preparing extracts of the plasma for bioassay. With the extract of plasma collected at night I can induce a response in the dermal melanophores of tadpoles indicating the presence of melatonin. With the extract of plasma collected during the day I cannot, indicating the absence of melatonin or concentrations below the sensitivity of the assay. Similarly, an extract of rat blood collected at night elicits the melanophore response while that prepared from blood collected during the day does not. Of course, such extracts are too crude to allow us to quantify the melatonin extracted or even be sure of its identity. We are presently attempting to refine the technique so that we can make such measurements.

DISCUSSION REFERENCES

Deguchi, T. and Axelrod, J. (1972). Proc. Natl. Acad. Sci. USA 69, 2208-2211.

Halberg, F., Haus, E., Cardoso, S., Scheving, L., Kühl, J., Shiotsuka, R., Rosene, G., Pauly, J., Runge, W., Spalding, J., Lee, J., and Good, R. (1973). Experientia 29, 909-934.

Lynch, H., Eng, J., and Wurtman, R. J. (1973). Proc. Natl. Acad. Sci. USA 70, 1704-1707.

Pelham, R. W., Vaughan, G. M., Sandock, K. L., and Vaughan, M. K. (1973). J. Clin. Endocrinol. Metab. 37, 341-344.

Weiss, B. (1968). Adv. Pharmacol. 6A, 152-155.

THE NEURAL AND HORMONAL BASES OF THE REPRODUCTIVE CYCLE OF THE RAT

R. A. Gorski, S. P. Mennin and K. Kubo

Department of Anatomy and Brain Research Institute
UCLA School of Medicine
Los Angeles, California 90024

OUTLINE

I. INTRODUCTION

The reproductive cycle of the female mammal is one of the most important biological rhythms. Through the coordination of vaginal, ovarian, pituitary, neuroendocrine and behavioral rhythms, reproduction and the propagation of the species is made possible. This reproductive cycle, which in large measure is a manifestation of the regulation of pituitary gonadotropin (GTH) secretion by the central nervous system (CNS), has several distinctive characteristics: 1) Although related to the daily light cycle, the period of the reproductive cycle is much longer, ranging from four or five days in the rat (which will be the principal species considered in this discussion), to the monthly cycle of the human.

Original research of the authors supported by NIH Grant HD-01182 and by the Ford Foundation.

2) Although clearly a manifestation of a neural rhythm, the normal expression of that rhythm is totally dependent on the feedback action of gonadal hormones. 3) Although this biological rhythm is sexually dimorphic, ontogenic studies have demonstrated that it is determined by the hormone environment at a critical period in development.

In the present discussion we will review the experimental evidence for several fundamental concepts of the hormonal and neural bases of the reproductive cycle in the female rat, as well as that for the sexual differentiation of the regulatory mechanisms involved. Upon this foundation, we shall then consider more recent data which may suggest modification of these concepts. Unfortunately, time and space will not permit extensive consideration of all the rhythmic processes which comprise the reproductive cycle. We will focus our attention on those events which lead to ovulation and the readiness to mate. Since sexual behavior reflects the functional state of rhythmic regulatory processes in the female just as does ovulation, both phenomena will be discussed.

II. BASIC CONCEPTS OF THE REGULATION OF THE REPRODUCTIVE CYCLE

The purpose of this section is to present a broad overview of current understanding of the regulation of the reproductive cycle. To accomplish this, the experimental evidence in support of this understanding will be outlined. Several points are well established, however, and space will not permit inclusive literature citations. When appropriate, individual papers will be cited but in many cases the interested reader will be referred to relevant detailed reviews.

1. Hormonal Basis of the Estrous Cycle

The rhythmic nature of the reproductive process in the female rat is clearly demonstrated by the temporal pattern of change in the plasma level of several hormones (Figure 1). The key event during this cycle is the release of a surge of luteinizing hormone (LH). In intact females housed under a controlled environment of 14 hours of light per day, plasma LH remains very low except for a brief period late in the afternoon of the day of vaginal proestrus. At this time there is a surge of LH secreted by the pituitary, and plasma LH levels increase by approximately ten-fold (Monroe, Rebar, Gay and Midgley, 1969; Gay, Midgley and Niswender, 1970; Brown-Grant, 1971). Follicle stimulating hormone (FSH) secretion also increases at this time. Studies that are now classical revealed that this surge of LH is brought about by the CNS (see Everett, 1969, 1970, 1972). In fact, the neural stimulus effective in releasing LH-Releasing Factor (LRF) to bring about the ovulatory surge of LH is restricted to a period of 30-45 minutes in individual rats. For an entire colony of animals, the release of LRF occurs during a relatively brief period (between 2-4 pm. for the inbred Osborne-Mendel strain). The importance of this event is embodied in the term "critical period" (Everett, 1969, 1970). The fact that ovulation can be delayed by units of approximately 24 hours by the repetitive injection of pentobarbital just prior to this critical period led to the general concept that the neural stimulus for the ovulatory surge of LH has at least the potential to exhibit a 24-hour periodicity (Everett, 1969, 1970).

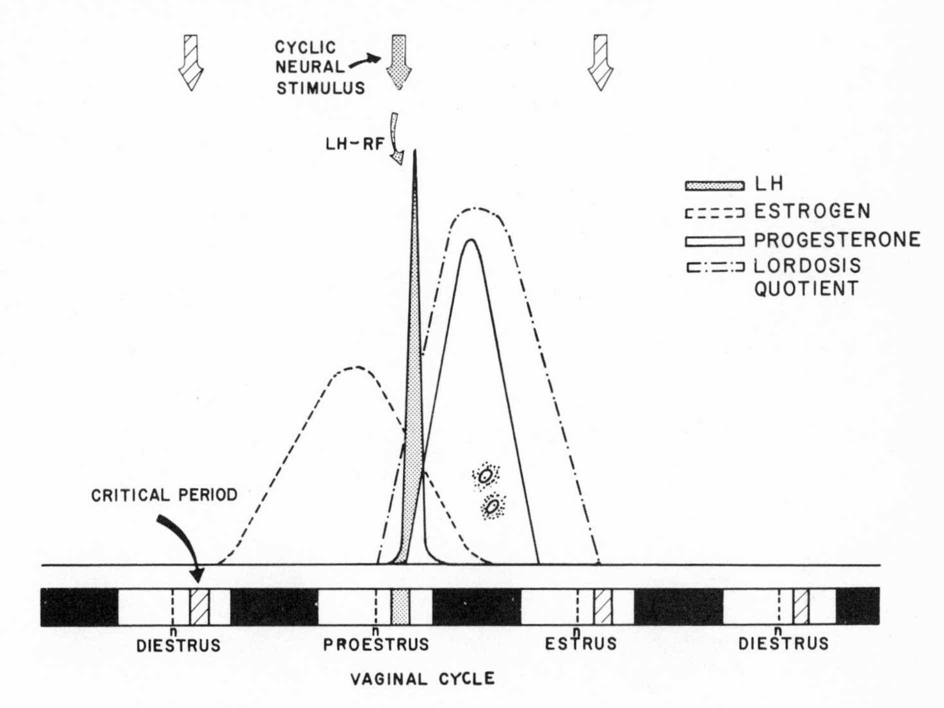

Figure 1. Highly schematic representation of the cyclic changes in plasma luteinizing hormone (LH), estrogen, and progesterone during the reproductive cycle of the female rat. Superimposed on these hormonal changes is a curve representing the rate of lordosis responding over this same time period as adapted from Hardy (1972). Reprinted from Gorski (1973a).

Although the cyclic release of the LH surge is the result of a rhythmic process within the brain, that process is dependent on the hormone environment. Following ovariectomy, plasma GTH levels increase markedly and reach high, apparently steady levels as determined by bioassay (McCann and Ramirez, 1964). However, more recent analyses using the sensitive radioimmunoassay (RIA) challenge this concept (see Section III. 2.). The absence of the cyclic release of GTH comparable to that of the intact rat was demonstrated for the spayed female in a clever, although indirect experiment (Takewaki, 1962). In the ovariectomized female, intrasplenic ovarian grafts become heavily luteinized in response to the high plasma titers of GTH, but the steroid hormones secreted in these ovarian grafts do not escape the hepatic circulation in quantities sufficient to inhibit GTH secretion. Takewaki (1962) implanted vaginal tissue adjacent to intrasplenic ovarian grafts and failed to find evidence of the cyclic secretion of ovarian steroids and thus, of GTH

(Figure 2). Whatever the source of periodicity of the neural stimulus for the ovulatory surge of LH, it appears to depend on hormonal feedback for its functional expression.

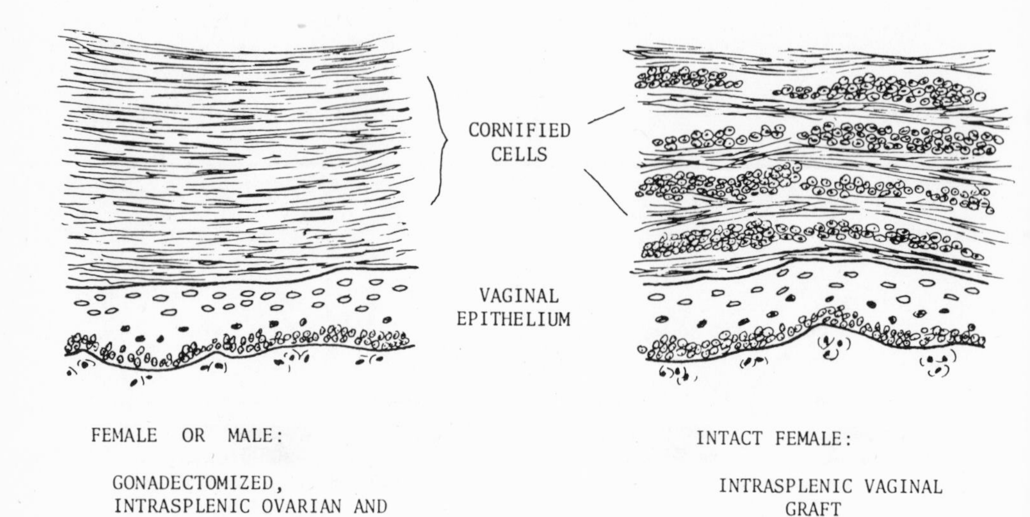

Figure 2. The pattern of pituitary gonadotropin release as indicated by the cytology of intrasplenic vaginal grafts in the intact female and in gonadectomized rats with intrasplenic ovarian grafts. Schematic diagram drawn from histological photographs from Takewaki (1962).

In this regard, estrogen is the hormone of most importance. In many mammalian forms including the rat, the surge of LH follows or coincides with a peak in endogenous estrogen secretion (Brown-Grant, 1971). Although careful study of Figure 1 might suggest that a fall in plasma estrogen actually triggers the surge of LH, it should be pointed out that sufficient estrogen to support the release of LH has already been secreted by 10 am on the morning of vaginal proestrus (Schwartz, 1969). It may be that the further secretion of estrogen is required to facilitate female sexual behavior, and/or possibly it ensures that a threshold level of estrogen is surpassed in order to "guarantee" ovulation. In several mammals estrogen clearly serves a facilitatory or positive feedback function (Davidson, 1969; Brown-Grant, 1971; Karsch, Dierschke, Weick, Yamaji, Hotchkiss and Knobil, 1973; also see Section III.3.).

Although exogenous progesterone can facilitate (or inhibit) ovulation when administered at specific times during the estrous cycle (Everett, 1969, 1970; Davidson, 1969; Brown-Grant, 1971; Brown-Grant and

Naftolin, 1972), the temporal pattern of endogenous hormone levels suggests that it is the release of pituitary LH which stimulates ovarian progesterone secretion and not the reverse (Barraclough, Collu, Massa and Martini, 1971). It may be that the increase in progesterone secretion is related to behavioral receptivity rather than to ovulation. In the rat, behavioral receptivity is another rhythmic neural process that is dependent upon gonadal hormones. The ovariectomized rat will not display sexual behavior, as defined by the lordosis reflex (Figure 3),

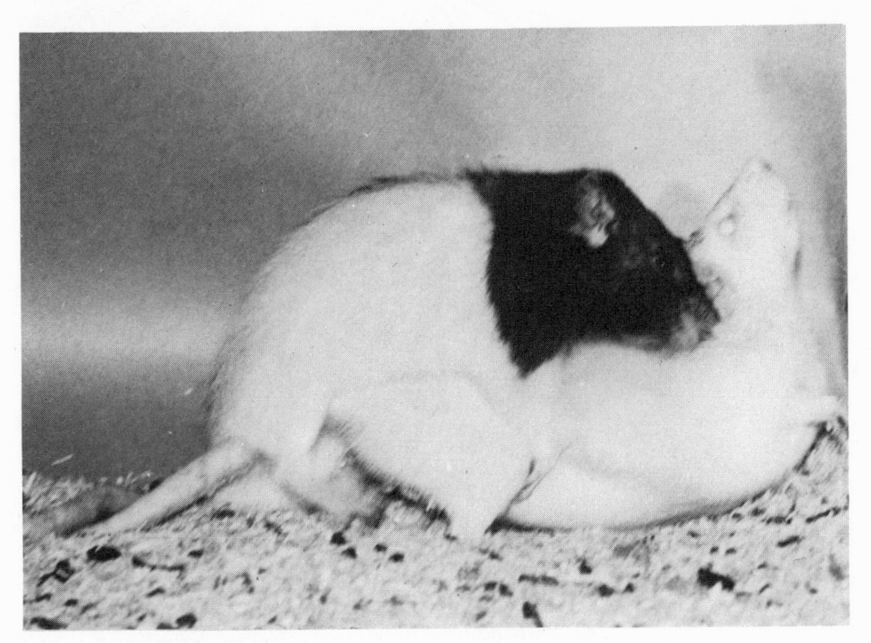

Figure 3. An example of lordosis behavior exhibited by the receptive female rat to the mounting activity of the male.

however, estrogen treatment alone can restore normal levels of lordosis behavior (Davidson, Smith, Rodgers and Bloch, 1968; Gorski, 1973a). Importantly, when more physiological doses of estrogen are administered, lordosis behavior is markedly and rapidly facilitated by progesterone (Edwards, Whalen and Nadler, 1968; Gorski, 1973a). Because of the relatively brief period of increased exposure of the brain to endogenous estrogen during the normal estrous cycle (Figure 1), it is probable that sexual behavior of the intact female is a response of the brain to the sequential exposure to both estrogen and progesterone.

2. Neural Basis of the Estrous Cycle

There is considerable experimental support for the view that the hypothalamic control of the release of hypophyseal LH can be divided into two fundamental levels (for extensive reviews see Flerkó, 1966; Barraclough, 1967; Everett, 1969; Gorski, 1971a). In general, the arcuate nucleus and surrounding area of the medial basal hypothalamus (MBH) is thought to contain neurons which regulate the tonic secretion of GTH (Figure 4). The MBH is a rich source of releasing factors. Elec-

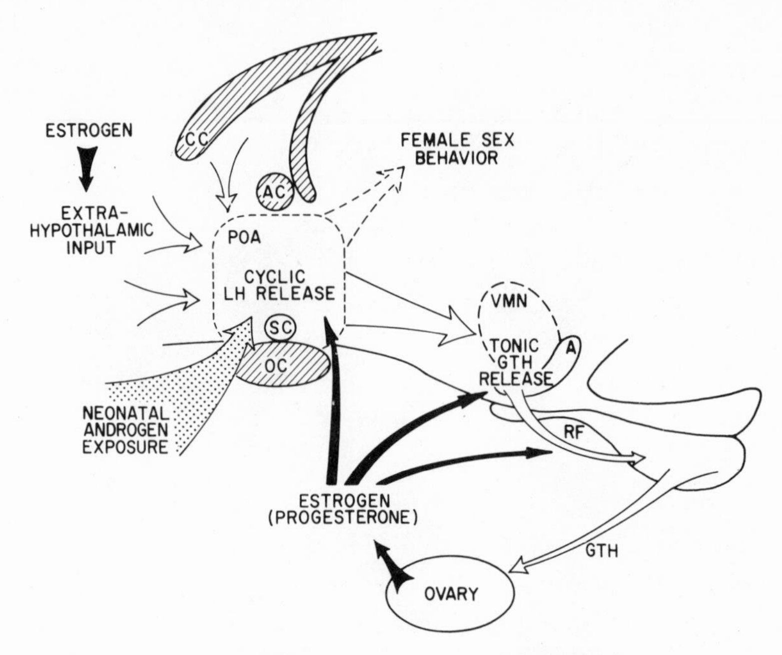

Figure 4. Localization on a schematic parasagittal diagram of the rat brain of the neural control of hypophyseal secretion. The solid arrows indicate estrogen or estrogen/progesterone feedback. Please see text for discussion. Abbreviations: A, arcuate nucleus; AC, anterior commissure; CC, corpus callosum; OC, optic chiasm; POA, preoptic area; RF, releasing factors; SC, suprachiasmatic nucleus; VMN, ventromedial nucleus. Reprinted from Gorski (1970).

trolytic lesions of this region suppress pituitary function and lead to gonadal atrophy. On the other hand, complete deafferentation of the MBH can result in a condition of anovulatory persistent vaginal cornification with polyfollicular ovaries. Interestingly, in some animals, deafferentation of the MBH results in persistent diestrus. No explanation for these different results is currently available. The development of anovulatory persistent estrus, however, suggests that the neurally isolated MBH can support the tonic secretion of GTH. LH release and even ovulation can be induced by applying electrical current or by depositing iron electrolytically in this region. Further evidence for the role of the arcuate region in the regulation of pituitary-gonadal function is provided by the observations that this region contains neurons which have an active estrogen uptake system and that estrogen implants result in gonadal atrophy.

The fact that spontaneous ovulation cannot occur after complete deafferentation of the MBH suggests that the neural stimulus for the cyclic surge of LH must arise outside of this area. The generally accepted hypothesis at the present time assumes that the preoptic-anterior hypothalamic area (POA-AHA) is an important integrative center for the LH surge, if not the site of origin of the neural stimulus responsible for this surge (Figure 4). The same experimental approaches as described above have also been applied to the question of the possible function of this area. Lesions in the POA-AHA prevent ovulation and induce a state of persistent vaginal estrus with polyfollicular ovarian development, whereas stimulation of this region can induce LH release and ovulation.

The functional effects of two experimental knife cuts are consistent with the presumed role of the POA in ovulation. As Halász and Gorski (1967) initially demonstrated, a knife cut placed in the retrochiasmatic area, thus transecting possible neural connections between the POA-AHA and the arcuate region, blocks ovulation and again induces persistent vaginal estrus and polyfollicular ovarian development. Subsequent studies (Köves and Halász, 1970; Kaasjager, Woodbury, van Dieten and van Rees, 1971) suggest that the POA-AHA can generate at least an occassional spontaneous surge of LH independent of its antero-lateral neural connections. The POA-AHA also contains neurons which bind estrogen, which suggests that this region of the brain may respond to changes in ovarian activity in support of its presumed critical role in ovulation. In addition, the POA apparently receives information about environmental righting directly through retenohypothalamic fibers (Moore, Karapas and Lenn, 1971).

Although Figure 4 indicates a key role of the POA-AHA in the regulation of ovulation, it also suggests that this region of the brain in turn may be modulated by extrahypothalamic structures. In fact, as will be discussed in Section III.4., there is no doubt that neural structures other than the hypothalamus can influence GTH secretion. The important questions are: Which specific areas of the brain are involved in GTH regulation? What is the nature of their role in the control of the reproductive cycle?

Since the preceeding questions cannot be answered completely at this time, current understanding of the neural control of GTH secretion is limited to the final common pathway: POA-AHA to arcuate region to the pituitary. In the case of sexual behavior, however, no final common pathway has been identified; behavior is a much more diffuse and complex function of the CNS than is the production of releasing factors. Therefore, at the present time it is not possible to present a simple concept of the neural regulation of sexual behavior. There is general agreement that estrogen acts at the level of the POA-AHA to facilitate the cyclic display of female sexual behavior (see Gorski, 1973a). However, the possible site of progesterone action is far more controversial.

The authors' laboratory has formulated a working hypothesis that in the female rat, progesterone acts at the level of the mesencephalic reticular formation (MRF) to facilitate lordosis behavior. This hypothesis is based on the observation that the direct application of progesterone to this region of the brain rapidly facilitates lordosis behavior (Ross, Claybaugh, Clemens and Gorski, 1971).

More recently we have also examined the influence of progesterone on the electrical activity of the MRF. Progesterone alters the spontaneous activity of single cells in the MRF when injected intravenously in the estrogen primed ovariectomized rat (Figure 5). Similarly, the

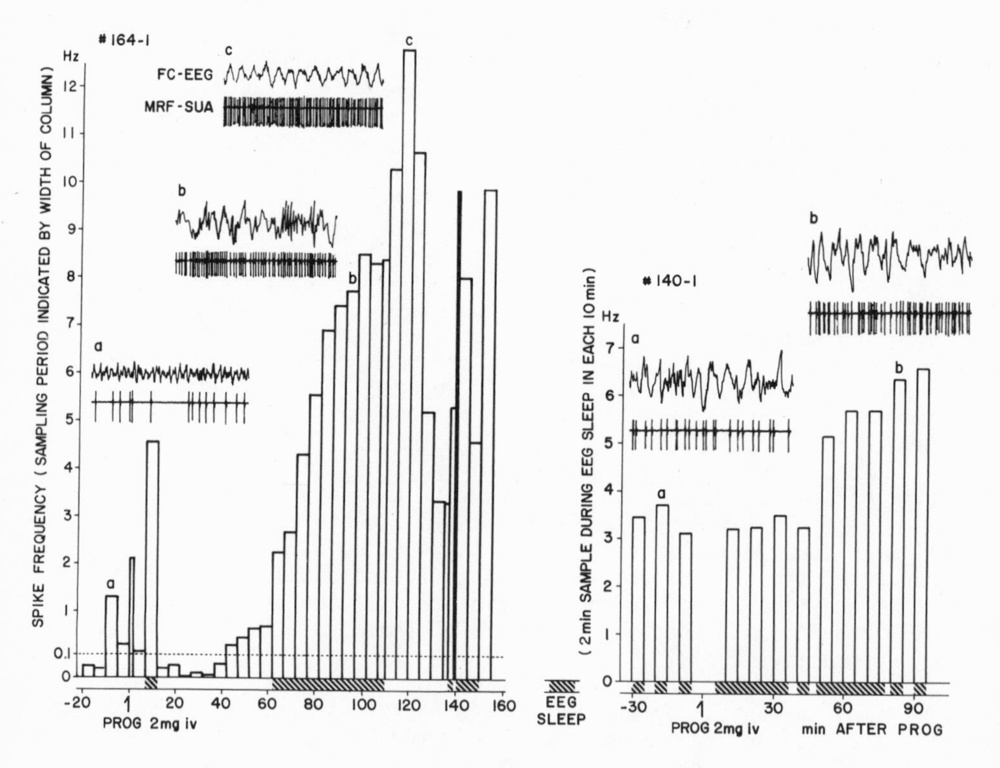

Figure 5. The effect of intravenous progesterone (aqueous suspension) injection on the electrical activity of two individual neurons in the mesencephalic reticular formation (MRF) of the estrogen-primed ovariectomized rat. The inserts present the EEG of the frontal cortex and spike discharges of the neurons obtained at the indicated positions on the spike frequency histogram of single unit activity (SUA) plotted against time after progesterone injection.

multi-unit activity of the MRF increases when crystalline progesterone is applied directly to this region (Figure 6). Progesterone adminis-

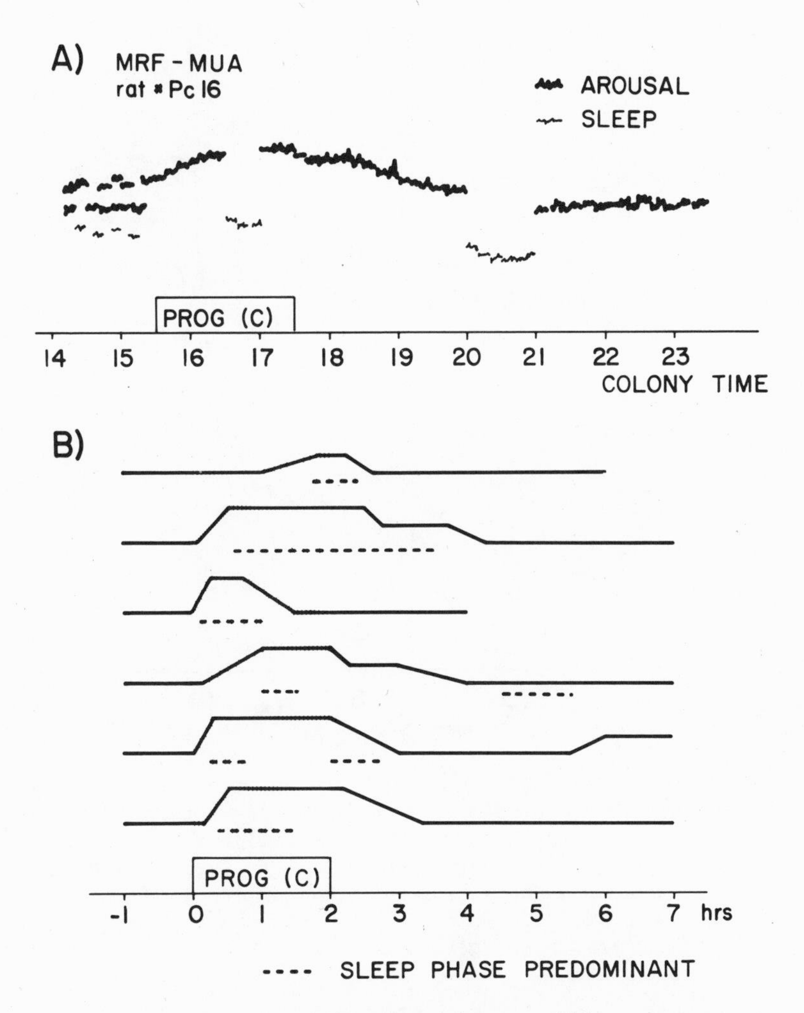

Figure 6. Influence of the application of crystalline progesterone [PROG (C)] to the mesencephalic reticular formation (MRF) on the multi-unit activity (MUA) recorded from the area of the implant. After a period of control recording of MUA, a progesterone-containing inner cannula was inserted in the MRF of estrogen-primed ovariectomized rats for two hours. A) The integrated MUA during cortical arousal and sleep for one rat. B) Schematic summary of the response in six animals.

tration also appears to facilitate the responsiveness of the MRF to sensory stimuli, particularly these related to genital stimulation (Figure 7). The possible significance of progesterone induced altera-

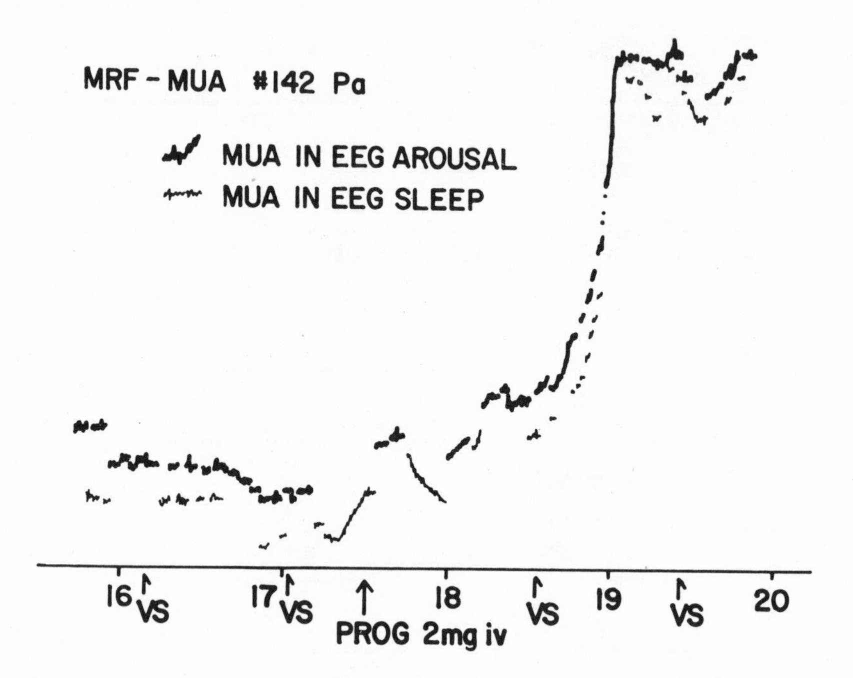

Figure 7. Facilitation of the integrated multi-unit (MUA) response of neurons in the mesencephalic reticular formation (MRF) to vaginal cervical stimulation (VS) following intravenous injection of an aqueous suspension of progesterone (PROG). Numbers indicate colony time. #142 Pa refers to rat number 142-progesterone, aqueous.

tions in the electrical activity of the MRF can be inferred from another series of experiments. Suppression of cerebral cortical function by the direct application of potassium chloride (Clemens, Wallen and Gorski, 1967; Clemens, 1971; Ross and Gorski, 1973) and electrical stimulation (Ross, Gorski and Sawyer, 1973), two procedures which induce cortical spreading depression, functionally replaces ovarian progesterone in the facilitation of lordosis behavior in estrogen-primed ovariectomized rats. Since the MRF regulates cortical activity, progesterone may facilitate sexual behavior by altering cortical function by a direct action at the level of the mesencephalon. This working hypothesis requires further experimental proof and at the present time it is difficult to formulate a simple concept to explain the behavioral rhythm which accompanies the estrous cycle.

3. Sexual Differentiation of the Hypothalamus

In the preceeding discussion we have purposely considered only the female since the regulation of reproductive activity in the rat is sexually dimorphic. In contrast to the female, the intact male displays essentially consistent gonadal and behavioral activity. Although diurnal fluctuations in hormone production and behavior may exist in the male, these are not comparable to the markedly rhythmic activity of the female. The concept of the sexual differentiation of the hypothalamus, however, states that this sexual dichotomy in hypothalamic function is not determined by a genetic difference in the brain, but rather is dependent upon the hormonal environment during a particular phase in development (for reviews see Barraclough, 1967; Gorski, 1971a, 1973b). In the rat, this phase encompasses the perinatal period. Several observations have established the fundamental aspects of this concept. With respect to the regulation of GTH secretion, the behavior of intraocular or subcutaneous ovarian transplants in males and females gonadectomized as adults illustrate the sex difference. Ovarian grafts luteinize cyclically in the female and support regular vaginal cycles. In the male castrated as an adult, however, similar grafts exhibit persistent cornification. On the other hand, if the male rat is orchidectomized within 1-3 days after birth and then given ovarian grafts as an adult, these grafts luteinize cyclically and support cyclic changes in vaginal graft cytology.

There is also a distinct sex difference with respect to the regulation of lordosis behavior. Male rats, orchidectomized when adult and primed with a regime of estrogen and progesterone effective in restoring lordosis behavior in the ovariectomized female, will rarely show a lordosis response to the mounting activity of stud males. In marked contrast, the adult male castrated within the first few days of life responds essentially as well as the female to estrogen and progesterone and a stud male by frequently exhibiting lordosis when mounted. Thus, the male rat castrated within the first few days of life exhibits functional characteristics normally associated with the female, e.g., the potential for the cyclic secretion of GTH and for the display of lordosis behavior. Because of these "female" characteristics, we have termed the neonatally castrated male the fale (for feminine male; Gorski, 1967). The functional differences between the fale and normal male demonstrate that the testes of the newborn rat secrete an agent which presumably changes hypothalamic function and permanently suppresses female regulatory patterns.

Although this important testicular substance has not been identified, exogenous testosterone propionate (TP) can apparently mimic its action to a degree in the neonatally castrated male and, importantly, in the intact female. Exogenous TP, when administered within approximately the first week of life in the female, permanently inhibits ovulation leading to a condition of persistent vaginal estrus and, according to the dose of TP, may also permanently suppress lordosis behavior. Even though it is unlikely that exposure of the developing brain of the female to TP exactly mimics the effects of testicular hormone in the male, this preparation, called the androgen-sterilized or androgenized female, has been studied extensively and productively. By using the female, the experimenter can control the site, onset, and duration of exposure to androgen as well as its dose. In addition, the ovaries of the intact female provide a convenient index of the pattern of GTH secretion. Thus, much of the experimental study of sexual differentiation of the brain, which occurs normally only in the male, has been carried out using the androgenized female preparation.

The concept of sexual differentiation of the hypothalamic control of GTH release is summarized schematically in Figure 8. At birth, the

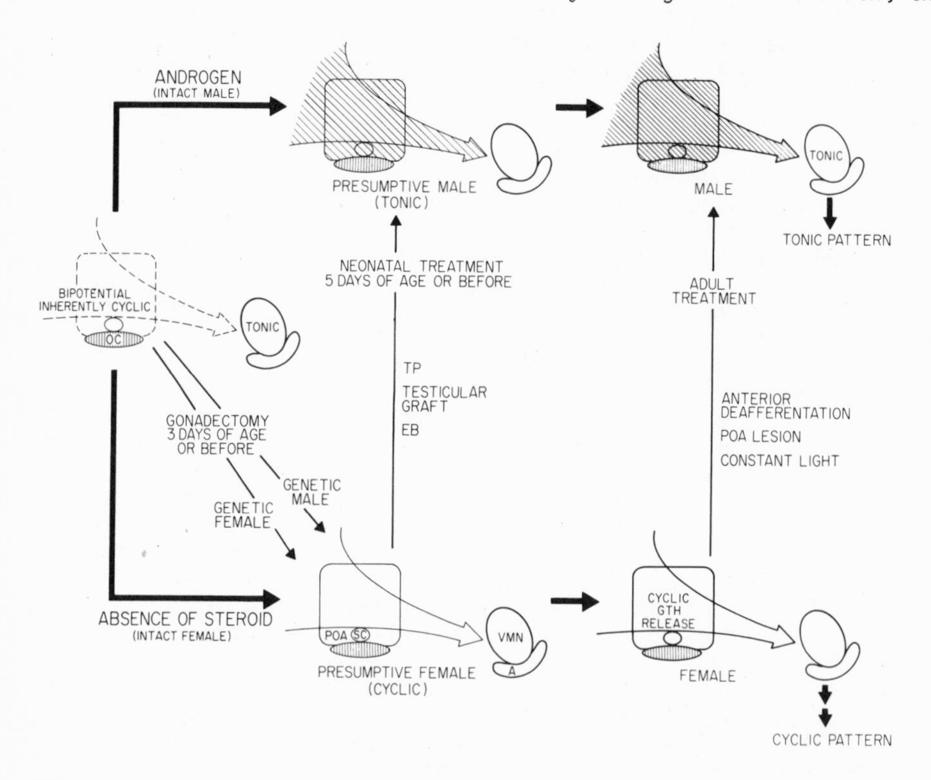

Figure 8. Schematic summary of the concept of the sexual differentiation of the neural control of pituitary gonadotropin (GTH) secretion in the rat. Please refer to text for discussion. Abbreviations: A, arcuate nucleus; EB, estradiol benzoate; OC, optic chiasm; POA, preoptic area; SC, suprachiasmatic nucleus; TP, testosterone propionate; VMN, ventromedial nucleus. Reprinted from Gorski (1971b).

POA-AHA is undifferentiated and essentially female. In the absence of affective levels of gonadal steroids (in the female and fale), this region develops fully its potential to regulate the cyclic surge of GTH provided a source of ovarian hormones is made available to the adult. However, if during this critical period of development, the hypothalamus is exposed to gonadal steroids (the intact male, or the female or fale injected with exogenous steroids) the cyclic regulation of GTH secretion is suppressed or fails to develop normally. In the adult fale, the neural substrate for the regulation of ovulation appears to be comparable to that of the female. Although it is not possible to suggest the site of action of androgen in suppressing lordosis behavior, the same general principle holds: if gonadal steroids act on the brain during this period of sexual differentiation, lordosis responsiveness is suppressed in the adult of either sex.

Note that Figure 4 includes reference to this concept of sexual differentiation of the hypothalamus and suggests that gonadal steroids can exert a permanent action on the developing POA-AHA during the neonatal period. In summary, this figure also illustrates the concept of the tonic and cyclic regulation of LH secretion. It is suggested that ovarian estrogen triggers the cyclic release of the surge of LH whereas ovarian progesterone, which is released in response to this surge, may play a role in facilitating sexual behavior. Although not shown in Figure 4, progesterone likely exerts its behavioral effect by an action at the level of the MRF. With these basic concepts in mind, we will now consider more recent data.

III. RECENT EXPERIMENTAL OBSERVATIONS AND THESE BASIC CONCEPTS

1. The Pituitary as a Site of Hormonal Feedback

Although Moore and Price (1932) originally proposed that the estrous cycle was regulated by a feedback action of ovarian estrogen on the pituitary gland, the gradual elucidation of the important role of the hypothalamus in regulating pituitary function shifted attention almost completely to the action of gonadal steroids on the hypothalamus. The existence of estrogen-concentrating neurons in the hypothalamus and elsewhere in the brain has been demonstrated (Eisenfeld and Axelrod, 1965; Kato and Villee, 1967; Pfaff, 1968; Stumpf, 1968, 1970; Anderson and Greenwald, 1969; for review see McEwen and Pfaff, 1973), and there currently is an active search for estrogen "receptor" macromolecules in the hypothalamus (Eisenfeld, 1970; Kato, 1973; and McEwen and Pfaff, 1973). Principally, because of the critical evaluation of the technique of direct application of steroids to the MBH by Bogdanove (1963), the possibility that gonadal steroids acted directly on the pituitary remained under consideration. More recent studies have strongly reinforced this possibility (Weick, Smith, Dominguez, Dhariwall and Davidson, 1971; Hilliard, Schally and Sawyer, 1971).

With the availability of synthetic luteinizing hormone releasing factor (LRF), however, this question has been convincingly resolved. Physiological fluctuations in ovarian hormone secretion significantly alter hypophyseal responsiveness to LRF. Rippel, Johnson and White

(1973) administered a large dose (5 μg) of synthetic LRF to intact cycling rats at 9 a.m. on each day of the vaginal cycle except estrus. They measured serum LH by radioimmunoassay (RIA) over the next several hours. Although LRF induced a significant release of LH at each stage of the estrous cycle, the amount released varied considerably. In response to the same dose of LRF, the proestrous female released approximately twice as much LH as did animals in diestrus or metestrus. Similarly, Nillius and Wide (1972) reported significant variation in the LH response to LRF with the stage of the human menstrual cycle.

The possible importance of this observation is illustrated by a recent study of Everett, Krey and Tyrey (1973). They report that the release of LH following electrochemical stimulation of the POA is significantly greater in proestrous rats than in animals in diestrus. As these investigators indicate, it is currently impossible to suggest whether this difference is due simply to varying hypophyseal sensitivity to LRF, changes in hypothalamic content of LRF, or as well, to a potentially important difference in central excitability. It has also been suggested that hypothalamic LRF is the releasing factor for both LH and FSH. Schally, Redding and Arimura (1973) use their observation of complex effects of sex steroids on the pituitary response to LRF *in vitro* to evaluate critically their suggestion that the steroid hormone environment at the level of the pituitary may determine the differential secretion of LH and FSH to the same releasing factor. Although consideration of this point in detail is beyond the scope of this discussion, it is evident that the feedback action of steroids at the level of the pituitary will play an important role in the elaboration of future concepts of the regulation of the reproductive cycle. The direct action of steroids on the pituitary may represent an important level of control of the estrous cycle, for some processes such as the differential secretion of LH and FSH; perhaps even more important than feedback at the neural level.

2. The Episodic Secretion of LH

Although we have indicated above that plasma GTH levels increase following gonadectomy to reach steady high levels, this concept is based on the bioassay of blood samples obtained at a frequency of once a day or much less. With the development of the sensitive RIA it became possible to measure GTH in small blood samples obtained from individual animals over a much shorter period of time. Impressed by apparently random but marked fluctuations in plasma LH in the ovariectomized monkey observed under these conditions, Dierschke, Bhattacharya, Atkinson and Knobil (1970) obtained very frequent blood samples and found that plasma LH concentration oscillated with a period of approximately one hour. This unexpected oscillation of plasma LH has been confirmed in many animals and it is now clear that LH is secreted in relatively brief episodes in the gonadectomized female (Figure 9) and male rat (Gay and Sheth, 1972), the ovariectomized ewe (Buttler, Malven, Willett and Bolt, 1972), and in both hypogonadal (Root, DeCherney, Russ, Duckett, Garcia and Wallach, 1972) and normal intact (Yen, Tsai, Naftolin, Vandenberg and Ajabor, 1972; Nankin and Troen, 1972; Kapen, Boyar, Hellman

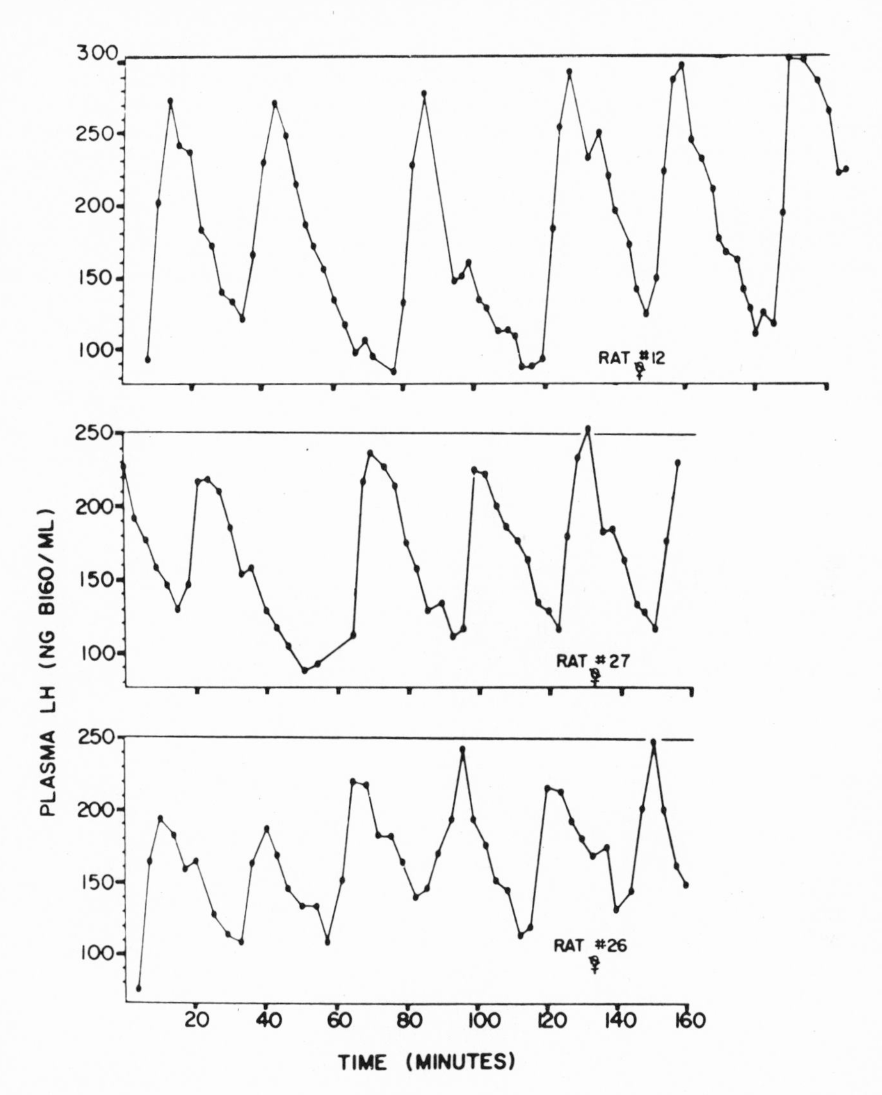

Figure 9. Episodic fluctuations in plasma luteinizing hormone (LH) concentration in untreated ovariectomized rats. Reprinted from Gay & Sheth (1972).

and Weitzman, 1973) humans. In fact, in the intact human many hormones are apparently secreted episodically (West, Mahajan, Chavre, Nabors and Tyler, 1973).

The physiological significance of episodic secretion of LH is unknown at the present time. Butler, Malven, Willett and Bolt (1972) have shown that at least in the ewe, episodic fluctuations in plasma LH are not due to peripheral changes in the metabolism of this hormone. The cranial output of LH (defined as the jugular venous concentration of LH minus carotid artery concentration) showed a similar oscillatory pattern. This observation suggests that LH is actually secreted episodically, but does not establish that this rhythm is due to an episodic secretion of LRF. This peculiar episodic pattern could be related to the secretory process itself in the very active pituitary gland of the gonadectomized animal.

If this episodic pattern of LH secretion is eventually proven to reflect the rhythmic secretion of LRF, it may be related to the feedback action of hypophyseal hormones, or perhaps it may reflect a rhythmic component of the so-called tonic GTH regulatory mechanism. Since episodic secretion of LH has been observed in both the female and male rat after gonadectomy (Gay and Sheth, 1972), its neural regulation probably will not be comparable to that which regulates the cyclic surge of LH in the female. In the intact human, oscillatory or episodic LH secretion has been seen to occur most frequently at night. Thus, episodic pituitary activity could be related to sleep and the underlying neural and neurotransmitter mechanisms. Although Rubin, Kales, Adler, Fagan and Odell (1972) reported an apparent relationship between the episodic secretion of LH and sleep in man, Boyar, Perlow, Hellman, Kapen and Weitzman (1972) failed to detect a similar relationship.

Finally, it is possible that the episodic secretion of LH represents a "technical artifact." For the purpose of introducing this concept, which has not been mentioned before in this conference, let us consider whether the episodic secretion of LH can have any affect on the gonad in the rat. Since in the rat episodic secretion of LH has been seen only after gonadectomy, it is difficult to study its effect on the gonad. However, the experiment of Takewaki (1962) which was discussed above provides an interesting model for consideration. As noted, Takewaki used the behavior of an intrasplenic graft of vaginal tissue adjacent to ovarian grafts to monitor the pattern of GTH secretion in the gonadectomized rat (Figure 2). Presumably GTH secretion under these circumstances would have been episodic, but the vaginal grafts provided no evidence of fluctuations in estrogen secretion. If the "physiological half-life" of the action of LH on the ovary in stimulating estrogen secretion exceeds the plasma half-life of LH, the intrasplenic ovarian graft might be expected to ignore the episodic pattern of LH secretion and respond only to an "average" level of plasma LH.

Obviously this interpretation must be qualified. The model of the intrasplenic ovarian-vaginal graft has limitations, and in fact, it could be that although the ovary does follow the episodic pattern of LH secretion, the vaginal epithelium may respond too sluggishly to reflect these oscillations. Although future experiments may reveal that the episodic secretion of LH is in fact significant, we bring up the problem of the "physiological half-life" of a hormone to ask this rhetorical question: Is it possible that the investigator's technical ability to measure fluctuations in some substances in the blood can actually surpass the ability of the biological system under study to detect these same changes?

3. Hormonal Feedback and the Timing of the Surge of LH

In the preceding consideration of the hormonal basis of the estrous cycle, we indicated that estrogen triggers the surge of LH, whereas progesterone is presumably more important for the facilitation of sexual behavior. However, it is well established that the administration of exogenous progesterone can promote the release of LH. In the present section, we will review this action of progesterone in more detail and suggest that adrenal progesterone may play an important role in spontaneous ovulation, and as well, that the cyclic surge can exhibit a clear diurnal rhythm.

In the intact female exhibiting a five-day estrous cycle, progesterone injected on the third day of diestrus advances ovulation by 24 hours (Everett, 1961). In the immature rat, exogenous progesterone can also advance by 24 hours precocious ovulation induced by pregnant mare's serum injection (Zarrow and Gallo, 1969). Progesterone administration can induce ovulation in rats rendered anovulatory by electrolytic destruction within the POA (Barraclough, Yrarrazaval and Hatton, 1964). In the ovariectomized rat primed with estrogen, progesterone treatment brings about a massive discharge of LH (Caligaris, Astrada and Tolersnik, 1968; Bishop, Kalra, Fawcett, Krulich and McCann, 1972). Finally, when progesterone is injected on the morning of proestrus, the neural stimulus for the surge of LH occurs several hours earlier than expected (Zeilmaker, 1966; Brown-Grant and Naftolin, 1972). These latter studies in particular suggest that the timing of the surge of LH is not unalterably locked to a 24-hour rhythm and that progesterone feedback can alter this timing. Coupled with the previous demonstrations of progesterone positive feedback, there is no doubt that progesterone can facilitate the surge of LH but does it normally do so? The failure to detect an increase in ovarian progesterone production until after the surge of LH has been initiated (Barraclough, Collu, Massa and Martini, 1971) was used above to suggest that ovarian progesterone normally facilitates sexual behavior rather than ovulation.

It is now apparent, however, that peripheral plasma levels of progesterone do increase in time to play a facilitatory role in normal ovulation (Barraclough, Collu, Massa and Martini, 1971; Brown-Grant, 1971; Feder, Brown-Grant and Corker, 1971). The source of this progesterone is the adrenal. Mann and Barraclough (1973) detected a diurnal rhythm of adrenal origin in plasma progesterone and reported that progesterone rises significantly before the critical period. It is possible that progesterone from this source plays a significant role in the spontaneous cyclic surge of LH in the normal rat. Presumably the marked increase in ovarian progesterone output following the LH surge is related to sexual behavior (Powers, 1970; Gorski, 1973a).

Studies of the positive feedback action of both progesterone and estrogen in the ovariectomized rat have also provided data which appear to confirm the existence of a diurnal rhythm in the surge of LH (Caligaris, Astrada and Talesnik, 1968; Taleisnik, Caligaris and Astrada, 1969; Caligaris, Astrada and Taleisnik, 1971; Bishop, Kalra, Fawcett, Krulich and McCann, 1972). To illustrate this point we shall refer to unpublished data from our laboratory. When either normal or androgenized adult female rats are injected with a large dose of estradiol benzoate (EB, 20 μg) several weeks after ovariectomy, there is a marked suppression of plasma LH for more than four days (data not shown, but see Caligaris, Astrada and Taleisnik, 1971). In contrast to this negative feedback effect, a second injection of 20 μg EB or 5 mg progesterone administered at noon colony time, 72 hours after the initial LH suppressing dose of EB, exerts a positive feedback action with a marked diurnal character (Figure 10). Plasma LH increases to, or above, pre-

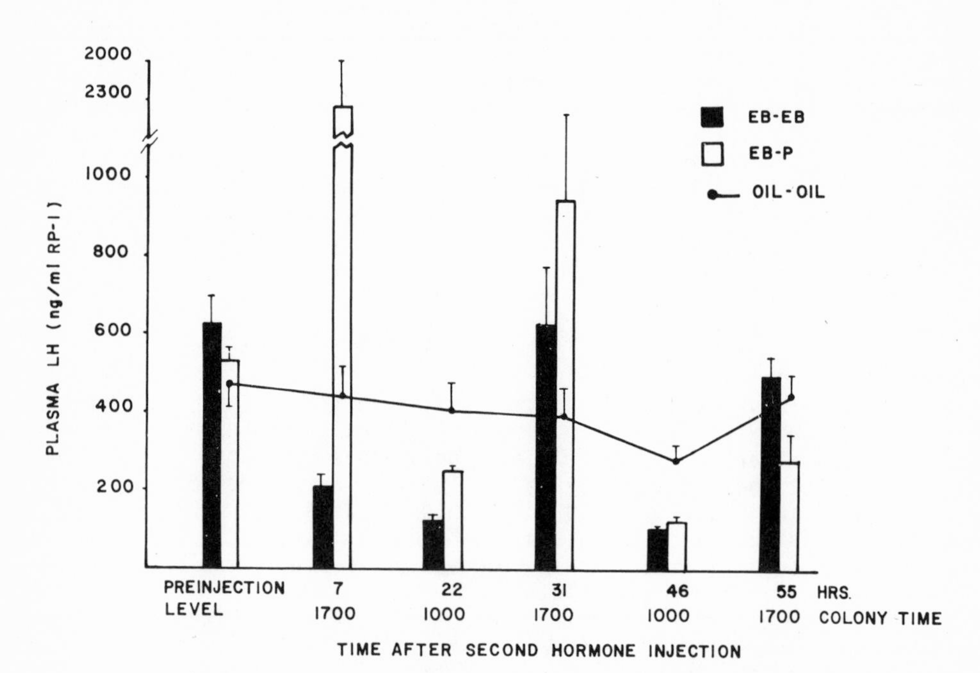

Figure 10. Effect of an injection of 20 μg estradiol benzoate (EB) or 5 mg progesterone (P) on plasma luteinizing hormone (LH) levels in ovariectomized normal rats treated 72 hours before with an LH-suppressing dose of 20 μg EB. The line graph indicates the levels of plasma LH in control ovariectomized rats receiving only oil. Note the afternoon peaks in plasma LH concentration.

injection postcastration levels during the afternoon but falls to low levels equivalent to those of estrogen suppressed animals in the morning. The response to progesterone is more dramatic and appears on the afternoon of hormone injection, approximately one day earlier than the

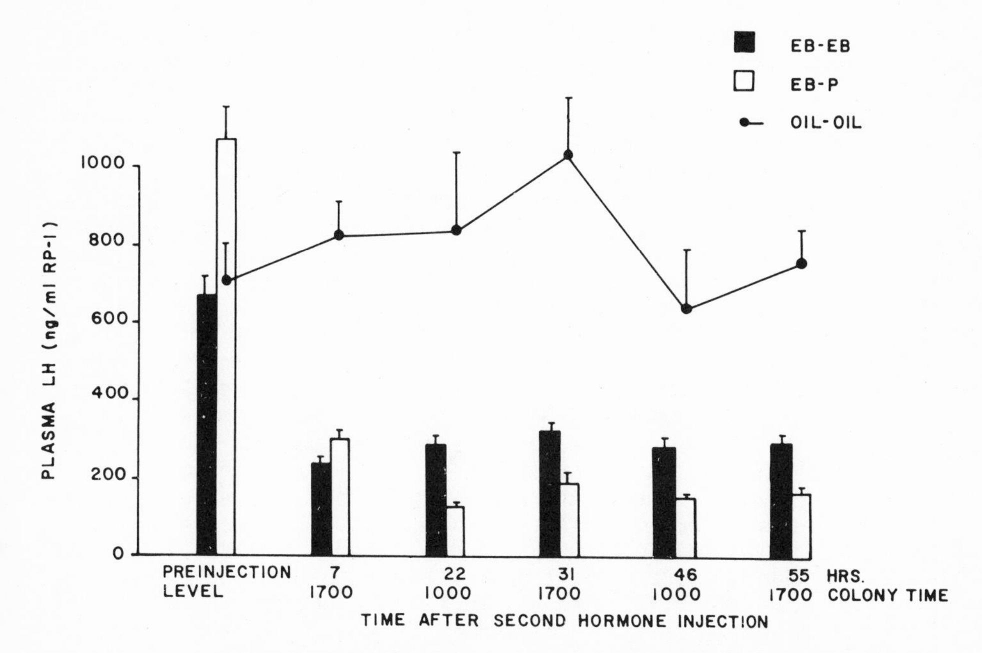

Figure 11. Effect of an injection of 20 μg estradiol benzoate (EB) or 5 mg progesterone (P) on plasma luteinizing hormone (LH) levels in ovariectomized androgenized rats treated 72 hours before with an LH-suppressing dose of 20 μg EB. The line graph indicates the levels of plasma LH in control ovariectomized rats receiving only oil. Note the absence of positive feedback.

response to the second injection of EB. As Figure 11 indicates, a positive feedback response to either estrogen or progesterone fails to occur in the ovariectomized androgenized female.

Although we did not determine the precise temporal pattern of this diurnal secretion of LH, it does appear to be related to the cyclic regulatory mechanism. In the androgenized female, in which the cyclic mechanism is thought to be non-functional, the hormone induced diurnal pattern of LH secretion is absent. If it can be determined that this diurnal pattern is independent of the adrenal rhythm in progesterone, these data would strongly support the concept that the neural stimulus for the LH surge has a periodicity of approximately 24 hours. In their classic studies Everett, Sawyer and Markee (1949) and Everett and Sawyer (1950) demonstrated that the LH surge had at least the potential to show a 24-hour rhythm provided the normal release of LH was blocked by administration of pharmacological agents. In the case of the present experimental design, LH was released in a surge-like manner on successive afternoons.

4. Extrahypothalamic Control of GTH Secretion

We have already suggested that extrahypothalamic structures can influence the regulation of the reproductive cycle (Figure 4). What areas of the brain have been shown to influence GTH secretion? How dependent is the hypothalamus on afferent input from these neural structures or systems? There is already an extensive literature in this area based on experiments utilizing the techniques of recording, stimulation, lesioning, drug administration, and hormone implantation (Gorski, 1973c). For the present consideration of biological rhythms it is important to recognize the dynamic role of extrahypothalamic structures in the regulation of the reproductive cycle. However, time and space limitations make it impossible to review this active area of research thoroughly. Therefore, only a few experiments of illustrative importance will be described.

The technique of electrochemical stimulation has been used extensively in the laboratory of Taleisnik to identify those neural structures which can markedly alter GTH secretion when activated. In animals exhibiting anovulatory persistent vaginal estrus because of exposure to continuous illumination, Velasco and Taleisnik (1969a) reported that acute electrochemical stimulation of the medial amygdala induced ovulation in 10 of 14 rats. However, when the stria terminalis, a major pathway from the amygdala to the hypothalamus, was transected, identical stimulation failed to induce ovulation in any of nine animals. When similar parameters of electrochemical stimulation were applied to the hippocampus exactly the opposite results were obtained (Velasco and Taleisnik, 1969b). In this experiment the hippocampus was stimulated just prior to the critical period on the afternoon of vaginal proestrus in normal cycling females. Such stimulation blocked spontaneous ovulation in approximately 80% of 24 rats. However, when the medial cortico-hypothalamic tract (an efferent pathway between the hippocampus and the MBH) was transected, hippocampal stimulation was much less effective in inhibiting ovulation. In a clever follow-up of their earlier study, these investigators also showed that hippocampal stimulation applied five minutes before electrochemical activation of the amygdala or the POA prevented the second stimulus from inducing ovulation in persistent estrous females. The observation that the hippocampus can inhibit LH release by means of impulses carried by the medial corticohypothalamic tract has been confirmed by Gallo, Johnson, Goldman, Whitmoyer and Sawyer (1971). On the other hand, Ellendorff, Colombo, Blake, Whitmoyer and Sawyer (1973) report that electrical stimulation of the amygdala can also inhibit ovulation.

In another series of experiments, Carrer and Taleisnik (1970, 1972) have mapped the mesencephalon and its ascending pathways in terms of the effect of their electrochemical activation on the release of LH. Stimulation of the ventral tegmental area of Tsai, medial raphe nucleus, periaqueductal gray, dorsal longitudinal fasciculus, or the caudal medial forebrain bundle just prior to the proestrous critical period in the normal rat suppressed ovulation. When Carrer and Taleisnik (1970) stimulated the dorsal mesencephalic tegmentum in the proestrous female, spontaneous ovulation was not blocked. However, when this dorsal tegmental (but not the ventral) area was stimulated electrochemically in the constant light exposed anovulatory animal, ovulation was induced. These investigators also measured the influence of stimulation of these various sites on plasma LH levels and found results generally consistent with their ovulation studies.

The cerebral cortex also appears to influence LH release. Taleisnik, Caligaris, and de Olmos (1962), and more recently Colombo and Sawyer (1973) have demonstrated that functional cortical inhibition (application of potassium chloride to the cortex) promotes LH release. Extrahypothalamic influences on pituitary activity are not limited to direct anatomical connections between neural systems and the hypothalamus since the pineal gland has been shown to inhibit LH release by means of a hormone, presumably melatonin (Reiter, 1972). In Figure 12, the

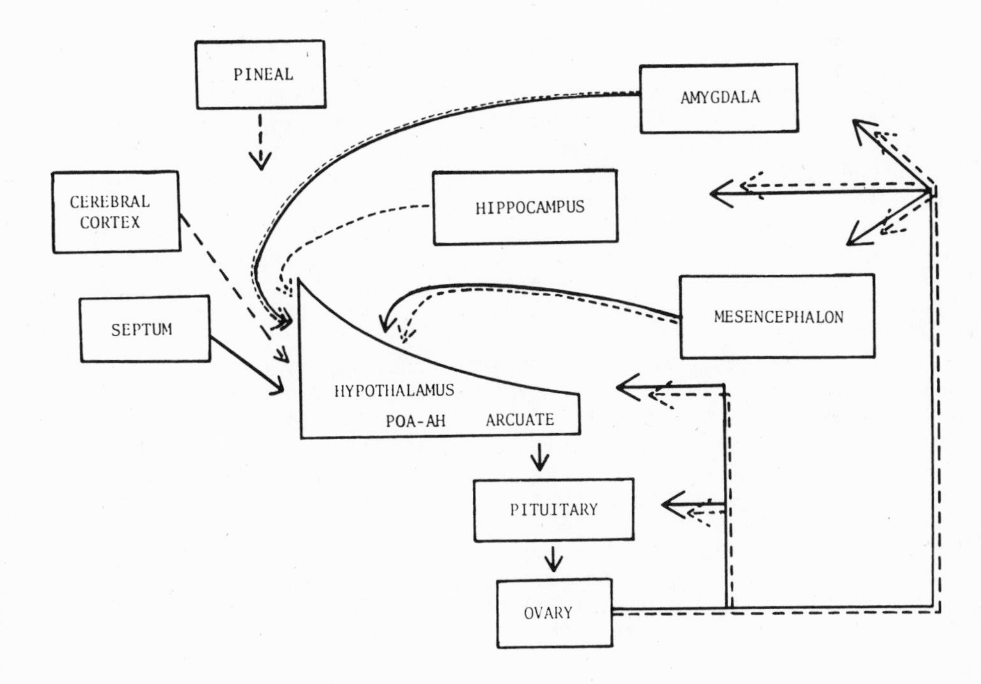

Figure 12. Schematic representation of structures which have been shown to have the potential to modify luteinizing hormone release. Solid lines represent facilitation, broken lines inhibition of LH release. Please see text for discussion of the evidence for this scheme.

various areas of the brain which have been shown to have the potential to facilitate or inhibit GTH release are illustrated schematically.

How dependent is pituitary function on influences from these areas? Is stimulatory input into the hypothalamus from the amygdala actually necessary for ovulation, for example? Transection of the stria terminalis (the pathway over which stimulatory input is apparently conducted to the hypothalamus) has only an acute inhibitory effect on ovulation (Velasco and Taleisnik, 1971). Following recovery from such surgery most of these animals resume normal ovulation. In fact, Köves and Halász (1970), and Kaasjager, Woodbury, van Dieter and van Rees (1971) have reported that ovulation can occur after antero-lateral deafferentation of the POA, thus it would appear that those extrahypothalamic structures which have been shown to alter GTH secretion modulate hypothalamic control systems. These extrahypothalamic structures appear to represent part of a highly complex and interrelated system of checks and balances which functions to ensure the appropriate regulation and timing of the reproductive cycle in terms of both the internal and external environment.

Although Figure 12 represents the facilitatory and inhibitory influences from various areas of the brain by means of arrows leading to the hypothalamus, this figure is not meant to imply a simple direct interaction between these structures and the hypothalamus. For example, Carrer and Taleisnik (1972) report that the inhibitory influence of mesencephalic areas on LH release can be mediated in part through the hippocampus-medial corticohypothalamic pathway. Not only are these extrahypothalamic structures interconnected through multiple and complex anatomical pathways, but an effect of steroid hormones on the brain may be to alter the functional "gain" of specific pathways (Kawakami and Kubo, 1971). The fact that steroids can act out of the hypothalamus is well documented (Stumpf, 1970; Ross, Claybaugh, Clemens and Gorski, 1971; McEwen and Pfaff, 1973).

It is clear that we cannot regard the ovulatory discharge of LH as the manifestation of a simple hypothalamic or preoptic neural "clock" independent of the rest of the nervous system. On the contrary, ovulation appears to be the result of the integration of a complex series of neural and hormonal influences, some facilitatory and some inhibitory, each perhaps with a rhythmic component to its function. It is possible that the POA carries out this important integrative function. Since the POA is hormonally responsive and may receive direct input from the retina, it might well have the ability to bring about the cyclic release of LH even after its antero-lateral neural connections are transected. In the normal animal, however, these complex connections play a critical role in hypothalamic function.

5. The Site of Sexual Differentiation of the Brain

One of the most interesting aspects of the regulation of reproductive activity is the sexual dimorphism of rhythmic function. As reviewed earlier in this discussion, it is generally held that exposure of the POA-AHA to androgen during a critical phase in development permanently suppresses its cyclic potential. The evidence for this concept, which generally has been obtained from study of the androgenized female, can be summarized by the following observations: direct exposure of the POA-AHA of the neonatal female to testosterone prevents ovulation in the adult (Wagner, Erwin and Critchlow, 1966; Nadler, 1968). Electrolytic destruction of the POA-AHA or a retrochiasmatic knife cut in the normal female blocks ovulation and induces a similar endocrine state of polyfollicular ovarian development and persistent vaginal cornification (Halász and Gorski, 1967). Electrical stimulation of the POA-AHA, which can induce ovulation in the normal female, is ineffective in the androgenized rat (Barraclough and Gorski, 1961). Finally, electrolytic destruction of the POA-AHA or exposure to constant illumination blocks the cyclic release of LH in both the male and female (Gorski, 1967). Considering the fact that gonadal steroids directly influence hypophyseal sensitivity to releasing factors, and that many extrahypothalamic structures regulate hypothalamic function, can one defend this simplistic interpretation of androgenization?

Several observations appear to challenge this concept. Tersawa, Kawakami and Sawyer (1969) reported that electrochemical stimulation of the POA of the androgenized female could induce ovulation as readily as similar stimulation of normal animals. Arai (1971) reported that stimulation of the amygdala, which was effective in inducing ovulation in the constant light exposed normal rat, failed to do so in the androgenized female or male. In addition, Kawakami and Terasawa (1972) suggest that the amygdala and hippocampus of the androgenized female, rather than the POA, may differ functionally from normal. Because of these observations we have initiated a series of experiments which, although still in progress, also appear to challenge the above concept.

Although many experiments have used ovulation as an index of LH release following brain stimulation, Segal and Johnson (1959) and Astrada, Caligaris and Taleisnik (1969) indicated that the ovary of the androgenized female is relatively insensitive to GTH. As indicated in Table 1, we have confirmed this observation, in fact, in our laboratory the ovary of the androgenized rat appears to require from 5-10 times more LH for full ovulation. Although the normal spontaneous release of LH may be much greater than actually needed for ovulation, there is no assurance that following stimulation of the brain of the androgenized rat the excess release of LH can overcome a 10-fold difference in ovarian sensitivity. Thus, we conclude that ovulation cannot be used as a precise index of neural responsiveness in the androgenized female.

Because of the potential effect of the constant exposure to estrogen, the pituitary of the androgenized female rat could also be refractory to LRF. Therefore, as a control for our stimulation studies, the response of the androgenized rat to synthetic LRF was evaluated. For stimulation studies in the cycling animal, spontaneous ovulation is first blocked by pentobarbital anesthesia. Therefore, the effect of LRF on the pituitary secretion of LH was determined in pentobarbital anesthetized normal and androgenized rats. As illustrated in Figure 13, the secretion of LH was comparable in both animals up to a dose of 100 ng LRF/100 g body weight. At the highest dose (500 ng/100 g) the response to LRF was somewhat delayed in the androgenized rat but LH appeared to

TABLE 1. THE OCCURRENCE OF OVULATION IN RESPONSE TO INTRAVENOUS LUTEINIZING HORMONE (LH) IN PENTOBARBITAL ANESTHETIZED NORMAL PROESTROUS AND ANDROGENIZED RATS.*

Dose of LH (NIH-LH-S18) μg/0.1ml Saline	NORMAL PROESTRUS		ANDROGENIZED	
	No. Ovulating / No. Injected	No. Tubal Ova	No. Ovulating / No. Injected	No. Tubal Ova
10			6/6	7.8 ± 1.2**
5	2/2	12	6/7	4.8 ± 0.9
2			3/7	3.7
1	6/6	7.5 ± 1.5	0/6	
0.5	0/6			
Saline	1/8	11	0/9	

Received 90 μg testosterone propionate on day 2-3 of life.

**Mean ± SE for ovulating animals.*

reach the same level in both preparations. On the basis of this evidence, which could be complicated by anesthesia and by the fact that LRF was administered as an intravenous bolus, we conclude that plasma LH levels following brain stimulation provide a reasonable estimate of neural responsiveness to that stimulus.

At this point we have electrochemically stimulated more than 200 rats at currents of 20, 40, or 80 μamps and have failed to detect any difference between androgenized and normal rats with respect to the time course and increment in plasma LH or the location of positive sites of stimulation in the POA and more anterior sites. Although it may be that even threshold electrochemical stimulation is totally non-physiological and masks potential functional differences in the hypothalamus, it is also possible that androgen acts at another or additional sites rather than at the level of the POA. Further studies are required, but at this point the precise site or sites of the androgenization of GTH regulatory mechanisms remains to be established.

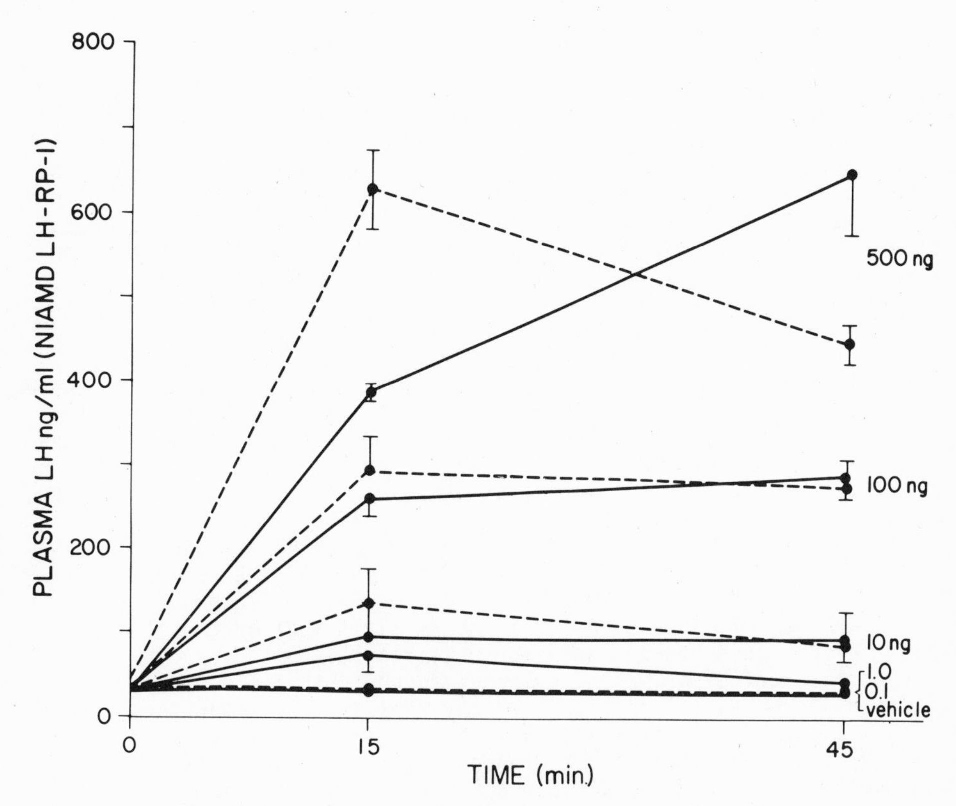

Figure 13. Influence of the intravenous injection of varying doses of synthetic luteinizing hormone releasing factor on the plasma concentration of luteinizing hormone (LH) in pentobarbital anesthetized androgenized rats (solid lines) and normal cycling rats on the afternoon of proestrus (broken lines).

Consideration of the androgenization of the regulation of lordosis behavior further emphasizes this fact. It is probable that the androgenized rat (male or female) is behaviorally less responsive to progesterone than is the normal female (Clemens, Hiroi and Gorski, 1969; Davidson and Levine, 1969; Clemens, Shryne and Gorski, 1970). As we have indicated above, it is possible that the site of action of progesterone in facilitating lordosis behavior is the MRF. Although still a hypothetical construct, it is possible that androgenization of the female rat includes a direct alteration in the hormonal responsiveness of the MRF.

IV. SUMMARY AND CONCLUSIONS

In the preceding discussion we have considered both the neural and hormonal control of a dramatic biological rhythm, the reproductive cycle of the female rat. In contrast to the rhythmic events in the female, the male exhibits only a tonic pattern of both pituitary and behavioral activity. This sexual dimorphism is determined shortly after birth in the rat with exposure of the developing brain to a testicular hormone, presumably androgen. The biological rhythm of the female, whether we refer to GTH release or lordosis behavior, is influenced in the adult by steroid hormone feedback, presumably upon steroid sensitive cells concentrated chiefly in the hypothalamus, but certainly not limited to this area. The neural regulatory substrate for the secretion of GTH appears also to be concentrated in the hypothalamus. The arcuate neurons which presumably produce releasing factors represent the last step in the final common pathway between the brain and the pituitary. More anteriorly, the POA-AHA appears to be critically important for cyclic GTH regulation. With respect to lordosis behavior, we cannot speak in terms of a precise final common pathway and it is difficult to formulate a simple concept of the regulation of behavior which might lead to experimental prediction, testing and modification. At the present time it would appear that estrogen acts in the POA-AHA, while progesterone may act in the MRF. The behavioral rhythm, like that of the cyclic secretion of LH, is dependent upon hormonal feedback.

More recent experimental evidence suggests that the direct feedback of gonadal hormones at the pituitary may represent an important level of control of the GTH rhythm since the local environment at the individual pituitary cell may determine the responsiveness of that cell to the hypothalamic releasing factors. Elegantly sensitive hormone assays now permit frequent sampling of blood even in small animals such as the rat and consequently allow a precise analysis of the temporal pattern of hormone release. At least in the gonadectomized rat, LH is secreted in brief episodes. It is possible that this episodic pattern is a reflection of the hypophyseal secretory process itself. In addition, one must at least consider the possibility that the scientist's ability to measure substances could theoretically exceed biological detection.

Several areas of the brain, including the cortex, amygdala, hippocampus, and mesencephalon have already been shown to be capable of modifying hypothalamic function, or at least GTH release. In addition, progesterone appears to act at the level of the MRF to alter behavior, perhaps through cortical mechanisms. Each of these systems may be found to have an intrinsic or imposed but independent neural rhythm. In addition, the pineal gland has a functional rhythm and the adrenal gland exhibits a rhythmic pattern of secretion including its production of progesterone which may contribute to the regulation or timing of reproductive events. There is also rhythmic photic input possibly directly into the POA, and there may be fundamental rhythms in the secretory process itself. All these biological rhythms may occur simultaneously. With rhythmic function so general, it is not at all surprising that GTH secretion and behavior are regulated cyclically. What is surprising is that out of the apparent chaos of these many mini-rhythms, a regular mega-rhythm, that of ovulation, occurs so consistently. Perhaps we should not look for the conceptual "ovulatory clock," but rather for a system which can integrate multiple rhythmic modulatory factors into a synchronized functional process. As a speculative hypothesis, we suggest that in the normal female rat the POA-AHA subserves this integrative function.

REFERENCES

Anderson, C. H. and Greenwald, G. S. (1969). Autoradiographic analysis of estradiol uptake in the brain and pituitary of the female rat. Endocrinology 85, 1160-1165.

Arai, Y. (1971). Effect of electrochemical stimulation of the amygdala on induction of ovulation in different types of persistent estrous rats and castrated male rats with an ovarian transplant. Endocrinology 18, 211-214.

Astrada, J. J., Caligaris, L., and Taleisnik, S. (1969). Ovulatory response induced by the injection of LH and/or FSH in normal and androgenized rats. Acta Physiol. Lat. Amer. 19, 291-295.

Barraclough, C. A. (1967). Modifications in reproductive function after exposure to hormones during the prenatal and early postnatal period. In: *Neuroendocrinology*, Volume II (Martini, L. and Ganong, W. F., eds.), pp. 61-99, Academic Press,-New York.

Barraclough, C. A. and Gorski, R. A. (1961). Evidence that the hypothalamus is responsible for androgen-induced sterility in the female rat. Endocrinology 68, 68-79.

Barraclough, C. A., Collu, R., Massa, R., and Martini, L. (1971). Temporal interrelationships between plasma LH, ovarian secretion rates and peripheral plasma progestin concentrations in the rat: effects of Nembutal and exogenous gonadotropins. Endocrinology 88, 1437-1447.

Barraclough, C. A., Yrarrazaval, S., and Hatton, R. (1964). A possible hypothalamic site of action of progesterone in the facilitation of ovulation in the rat. Endocrinology 75, 838-845.

Bishop, W., Kalra, P. S., Fawcett, C. P., Krulich, L., and McCann, S. M. (1972). The effects of hypothalamic lesions on the release of gonadotropins and prolactin in response to estrogen and progesterone treatment in female rats. Endocrinology 91, 1404-1410.

Bogdanove, E. M. (1963). Direct gonad-pituitary feedback: an analysis of effects of intracranial estrogenic depots on gonadotrophin secretion. Endocrinology 73, 696-712.

Boyar, R., Perlow, M., Hellman, L., Kapen, S., and Weitzman, E. (1972). Twenty-four hour pattern of luteinizing hormone secretion in normal men with sleep stage recording. J. Clin. Endocrinol. Metab. 35, 73-80.

Brown-Grant, K. (1971). The role of steroid hormones in the control of gonadotropin secretion in adult female mammals. In: *Steroid Hormones and Brain Function*, UCLA Forum Med. Sci. No. 15 (Sawyer, C. H. and Gorski, R. A., eds.), pp. 269-284, University of California Press, Los Angeles.

Brown-Grant, K. and Naftolin, F. (1972). Facilitation of luteinizing hormone secretion in the female rat by progesterone. J. Endocrinol. 53, 37-46.
Butler, W. R., Malven, P. V., Willett, L. B., and Bolt, D. J. (1972). Patterns of pituitary release and cranial output of LH and prolactin in ovariectomized ewes. Endocrinology 91, 793-801.
Caligaris, L., Astrada, J. J., and Taleisnik, S. (1968). Stimulating and inhibiting effects of progesterone on the release of luteinizing hormone. Acta Endocrinol. (Copenhagen) 59, 117-185.
Caligaris, L., Astrada, J. J.,, and Taleisnik, S. (1971). Release of luteinizing hormone induced by estrogen injection into ovariectomized rats. Endocrinology 88, 810-815.
Carrer, H. F. and Taleisnik, S. (1970). Effect of mesencephalic stimulation on the release of gonadotropins. J. Endocrinol. 48, 527-539.
Carrer, H. F. and Taleisnik, S. (1972). Neural pathways associated with the mesencephalic inhibitory influence on gonadotropin secretion. Brain Res. 38, 299-313.
Clemens, L. G. (1971). Perinatal hormones and the modification of adult behavior. In: *Steroid Hormones and Brain Function* (Sawyer, C. H. and Gorski, R. A., eds.), pp. 203-209, University of California Press, Los Angeles.
Clemens, L. G., Hiroi, M., and Gorski, R. A. (1969). Induction and facilitation of female mating behavior in rats treated neonatally with low doses of testosterone propionate. Endocrinology 84, 1430-1438.
Clemens, L. G., Shryne, J., and Gorski, R. A. (1970). Androgen and development of progesterone responsiveness in male and female rats. Physiol. Behav. 5, 673-678.
Clemens, L. G., Wallen, K., and Gorski, R. A. (1967). Mating behavior: Facilitation in the female rat following cortical application of potassium chloride. Science 157, 1208-1209.
Colombo, J. A. and Sawyer, C. H. (1973). Plasma LH changes following cortical spreading depression in female rats. Endocrinology 93, 182-187.
Davidson, J. M. (1969). Feedback control of gonadotropin secretion. In: *Frontiers in Neuroendocrinology* (Ganong, W. F. and Martini, L., eds.), pp. 343-388, Oxford University Press, New York.
Davidson, J. M. and Levine, S. (1969). Progesterone and heterotypical sexual behavior in male rats. J. Endocrinol. 44, 129-130.
Davidson, J. M., Smith, E. R., Rodgers, C. H., and Bloch, G. J. (1968). Relative thresholds of behavioral and somatic responses to estrogen. Physiol. Behav. 3, 227-229.
Dierschke, D. J., Bhattacharya, A. N., Atkinson, L. E., and Knobil, E. (1970). Circhoral oscillations of plasma LH levels in the ovariectomized Rhesus monkey. Endocrinology 87, 850-853.
Edwards, D. A., Whalen, R. E., and Nadler, R. D. (1968). Induction of estrus: estrogen-progesterone interactions. Physiol. Behav. 3, 29-33.
Eisenfeld, A. J. (1970). ^{3}H-Estradiol: In vitro binding to macromolecules from the rat hypothalamus, anterior pituitary and uterus. Endocrinology 86, 1313-1318.

Eisenfeld, A. J. and Axelrod, J. (1965). Selectivity of estrogen distribution in tissues. J. Pharmacol. Exp. Ther. 150, 469-475.
Ellendorff, F., Colombo, J. A., Blake, C. A., Whitmoyer, D. I., and Sawyer, C. H. (1973). Effects of electrical stimulation of the amygdala on gonadotropin release and ovulation in the rat. Proc. Soc. Exp. Biol. Med. 142, 417-420.
Everett, J. W. (1961). The mammalian female reproductive cycle and its controlling mechanisms. In: *Sex and Internal Secretions*, Volume 1 (Young, W. C., ed.), pp. 497-555, Williams & Wilkins, Baltimore, Maryland.
Everett, J. W. (1969). Neuroendocrine aspects of mammalian reproduction. Annu. Rev. Physiol. 31, 383-416.
Everett, J. W. (1970). Photoregulation of the ovarian cycle in the rat. Colloq. Int. Centre Nat. Rech. Sci. 172, 388-401.
Everett, J. W. (1972). The third annual Carl G. Hartman lecture: Brain, pituitary gland, and the ovarian cycle. Biol. Reprod. 6, 3-12.
Everett, J. W. and Sawyer, C. H. (1950). A 24-hour periodicity in the "LH-release apparatus" of female rats, disclosed by barbiturate sedation. Endocrinology 47, 198-218.
Everett, J. W., Sawyer, C. H., and Markee, J. E. (1949). A neurogenic timing factor in control of the ovulating discharge of luteinizing hormone in the cyclic rat. Endocrinology 44, 234-250.
Everett, J. W., Krey, L. C., and Tyrey, L. (1973). The quantitative relationship between electrochemical preoptic stimulation and LH release in proestrous versus late-diestrous rats. Endocrinology 93, 947-953.
Feder, H. H., Brown-Grant, K., and Corker, C. S. (1971). Pre-ovulatory progesterone, the adrenal cortex, and the "critical period" for luteinizing hormone release in rats. J. Endocrinol. 50, 29-39.
Flerkó, B. (1966). Control of gonadotropin secretion in the female. In: *Neuroendocrinology*, Volume I (Martini, L. and Ganong, W. F., eds.), pp. 613-618, Academic Press, New York.
Gallo, R. V., Johnson, J. H., Goldman, B. D., Whitmoyer, D. I., and Sawyer, C. H. (1971). Effects of electrochemical stimulation of the ventral hippocampus on hypothalamic electrical activity and pituitary gonadotropin secretion in female rats. Endocrinology 89, 704-713.
Gay, V. L. and Sheth, N. A. (1972). Evidence for a periodic release of LH in castrated male and female rats. Endocrinology 90, 158-162.
Gay, V. L., Midgley, A. R., Jr., and Niswender, G. D. (1970). Patterns of gonadotrophin secretion associated with ovulation. Fed. Proc. 29, 1880-1887.
Gorski, R. A. (1967). Localization of the neural control of luteinization in the feminine male rat (FALE). Anat. Rec. 157, 63-69.
Gorski, R. A. (1970). Localization of hypothalamic regulation of pituitary function. Amer. J. Anat. 129, 219-222.
Gorski, R. A. (1971a). Gonadal hormones and the perinatal development of neuroendocrine function. In: *Frontiers in Neuroendocrinology* (Martini, L. and Ganong, W. F., eds.), pp. 237-290, Oxford University Press, New York.

Gorski, R. A. (1971b). Steroid hormones and brain function: progress, principles and problems. In: *Steroid Hormones and Brain Function* (Sawyer, C. H. and Gorski, R. A., eds.), pp. 1-26, University of California Press, Los Angeles.

Gorski, R. A. (1973a). The neuroendocrine regulation of sexual behavior. In: *Advances in Psychobiology*, Volume II (Riesen, A. H., ed.), John Wiley and Sons, New York.

Gorski, R. A. (1973b). Perinatal effects of sex steroids on brain development and function. In: *Drug Effects on Neuroendocrine Regulation* (Gispen, W. H. and Zimmermann, E., eds.), Prog. in Brain

Gorski, R. A. (1973c). Extrahypothalamic influences on gonadotropin regulation. In: *The Control of the Onset of Puberty* (Grumback, M., Grace, G., and Mayer, F., eds.), in press, John Wiley and Sons, Inc., New York.

Halász, B. and Gorski, R. A. (1967). Gonadotrophic hormone secretion in female rats after partial or total interruption of neural afferents to the medial basal hypothalamus. Endocrinology 80, 608-622.

Hardy, D. F. (1972). Sexual behavior in continuously cycling rats. Behaviour 41, 288-297.

Hilliard, J., Schally, A. V. and Sawyer, C. H. (1971). Progesterone blockade of the ovulatory response to intrapituitary infusion of LH-RH in rabbits. Endocrinology 88, 730-736.

Kaasjager, W. A., Woodbury, D. M., van Dieten, J. A. M. J., and van Rees, G. P. (1971). The role played by the preoptic region and the hypothalamus in spontaneous ovulation and ovulation induced by progesterone. Neuroendocrinology 7, 54-64.

Kapen, S., Boyar, R., Hellman, L., and Weitzman, E. D. (1973). Episodic release of luteinizing hormone at mid-menstrual cycle in normal women. J. Clin. Endocrinol. Metab. 36, 724-728.

Karsch, F. J., Dierschke, D. J., Weick, R. F., Yamaji, T., Hotchkiss, J., and Knobil, E. (1973). Positive and negative feedback control by estrogen of luteinizing hormone secretion in the Rhesus monkey. Endocrinology 92, 799-804.

Kato, J. (1973). Localization of oestradiol receptors in the rat hypothalamus. Acta Endocrinol. (Copenhagen) 72, 663-670.

Kata, J. and Villee, C. A. (1967). Preferential uptake of estradiol by the anterior hypothalamus of the rat. Endocrinology 80, 567-575.

Kawakami, M. and Kubo, K. (1971). Neuro-correlate of limbic-hypothalamic-pituitary-gonadal axis in the rat: Change in limbic-hypothalamic unit activity induced by vaginal and electrical stimulation. Neuroendocrinology 7, 65-89.

Kawakami, M. and Terasawa, E. (1972). A possible role of the hippocampus and the amygdala in the androgenized rat: Effect of electrical or electrochemical stimulation of the brain on gonadotropin secretion. Endocrinol. Jap. 19, 349-358.

Köves, K. and Halász, B. (1970). Location of the neural structures triggering ovulation in the rat. Neuroendocrinology 6, 180-193.

Mann, D. R. and Barraclough, C. A. (1973). Changes in peripheral plasma progesterone during the rat 4-day estrous cycle: an adrenal diurnal rhythm. Proc. Soc. Exp. Biol. Med. 142, 1226-1229.

McCann, S. M. and Ramirez, V. D. (1964). The neuroendocrine regulation of hypophyseal luteinizing hormone secretion. Recent Prog. Horm. Res. 20, 131-170.

McEwen, B. S. and Pfaff, D. W. (1973). Chemical and physiological approaches to neuroendocrine mechanisms: attempts at integration. In: *Frontiers in Neuroendocrinology* (Ganong, W. F. and Martini, L., eds.), pp. 267-335, Oxford University Press, New York.

Monroe, S. E., Rebar, R. W., Gay, V. L., and Midgley, A. R., Jr. (1969). Radioimmunoassay determination of luteinizing hormone during the estrous cycle of the rat. Endocrinology 85, 720-724.

Moore, C. R. and Price, D. (1932). Gonad hormone functions, and the reciprocal influence between gonads and hypophysis with its bearing on the problem of sex hormone antagonism. Am. J. Anat. 50, 13-72.

Moore, R. Y., Karapas, F. and Lenn, N. J. (1971). A retino-hypothalamic projection in the rat. Anat. Rec. 169, 382-383.

Nadler, R. D. (1968). Masculinization of female rats by intracranial implantation of androgen in infancy. J. Comp. Physiol. Psychol. 66, 157-167.

Nankin, H. R. and Troen, P. (1972). Overnight patterns of serum luteinizing hormone in normal men. J. Clin. Endocrinol. Metab. 35, 705-709.

Nillius, S. J. and Wide, L. (1972). Variation in LH and FSH response to LH-releasing hormone during the menstrual cycle. J. Obstet. Gynaecol. Brit. Common. 79, 865-872.

Pfaff, D. W. (1968). Uptake of estradiol-17B-H^3 in the female rat brain. An autoradiographic study. Endocrinology 82, 1149-1155.

Powers, J. B. (1970). Hormonal control of sexual receptivity during the estrous cycle of the rat. Physiol. Behav. 5, 831-835.

Reiter, R. J. (1972). The role of the pineal in reproduction. In: *Reproductive Biology* (Balin, H. and Glasser, S., eds.), pp. 71-114, Excerpta Medica, Amsterdam.

Rippel, R. H., Johnson, E. S., and White, W. F. (1973). Ovulation and serum luteinizing hormone in the cycling rat following administration of gonadotropin releasing hormone. Proc. Soc. Exp. Biol. Med. 143, 55-58.

Root, A., DeCherney, A., Russ, D., Duckett, G., Garcia, C. R., and Wallach, E. (1972). Episodic secretion of luteinizing and follicle-stimulating hormones in agonadal and hypogonadal adolescents and adults. J. Clin. Endocrinol. Metab. 35, 700-704.

Ross, J. W. and Gorski, R. A. (1973). Effects of potassium chloride on sexual behavior and the cortical EEG in the ovariectomized rat. Physiol. Behav. 10, 643-646.

Ross, J., Claybaugh, C., Clemens, L. G., and Gorski, R. A. (1971). Short latency induction of estrous behavior with intracerebral gonadal hormones in ovariectomized rats. Endocrinology 89, 32-38.

Ross, J. W., Gorski, R. A., and Sawyer, C. H. (1973). Effects of cortical stimulation on estrous behavior in estrogen-primed ovariectomized rats. Endocrinology 93, 20-25.

Rubin, R. T., Kales, A., Adler, R., Fagan, T., and Odell, W. (1972). Gonadotropin secretion during sleep in normal adult male. Science 175, 196-198.

Schally, A. V., Redding, T. W., and Arimura, A. (1973). Effect of sex steroids on pituitary responses to LH- and FSH-releasing hormone in vitro. Endocrinology 93, 893-902.
Schwartz, N. B. (1969). A model for the regulation of ovulation in the rat. Recent Prog. Horm. Res. 25, 1-43.
Segal, S. J. and Johnson, D. C. (1959). Inductive influence of steroid hormones on the neural system: ovulation controlling mechanisms. Arch. Anat. Microsc. Morphol. Exp. 48 (Suppl.), 261-274.
Stumpf, W. E. (1968). Estradiol-concentrating neurons: topography in the hypothalamus by dry-mount autoradiography. Science 162, 1001-1003.
Stumpf, W. E. (1970). Estrogen-neurons and estrogen-neuron systems in the periventricular brain. Amer. J. Anat. 129, 207-218.
Takewaki, K. (1962). Some experiments on the control of hypophyseal-gonadal system in the rat. Gen. Comp. Endocrinol. Suppl. 1), 309-315.
Taleisnik, S., Caligaris, L., and Astrada, J. J. (1969). Sex difference in the release of luteinizing hormone evoked by progesterone. J. Endocrinol. 44, 313-321.
Taleisnik, S., Caligaris, L., and de Olmos, J. (1962). Luteinizing hormone release by cerebral cortex stimulation in rats. Amer. J. Physiol. 203, 1109-1112.
Terasawa, E., Kawakami, M., and Sawyer, C. H. (1969). Induction of ovulation by electrochemical stimulation in androgenized and spontaneously constant-estrous rats. Proc. Soc. Exp. Biol. Med. 132, 497-501.
Velasco, M. E. and Taleisnik, S. (1969a). Release of gonadotropins induced by amygdaloid stimulation in the rat. Endocrinology 84, 132-139.
Velasco, M. E. and Taleisnik, S. (1969b). Effect of hippocampal stimulation on the release of gonadotropin. Endocrinology 85, 1154-1159.
Velasco, M. E. and Taleisnik, S. (1971). Effects of interruption of amygdaloid and hippocampal afferents to the medial hypothalamus on gonadotrophin release. J. Endocrinol. 51, 41-55.
Wagner, J. W., Erwin, W., and Critchlow, V. (1966). Androgen sterilization produced by intracerebral implants of testosterone in neonatal female rats. Endocrinology 79, 1135-1142.
Weick, R. F., Smith, E. R., Dominguez, R., Dhariwal, A. P. S., and Davidson, J. M. (1971). Mechanism of stimulatory feedback effect of estradiol benzoate on the pituitary. Endocrinology 88, 293-301.
West, C. D., Mahajan, D. K., Chavre, V. J., Nabors, C. J., and Tyler, F. H. (1973). Simultaneous measurement of multiple plasma steroids by radioimmunoassay demonstrating episodic secretion. J. Clin. Endocrinol. Metab. 36, 1230-1236.
Yen, S. S. C., Tsai, C. C., Naftolin, F., Vandenberg, G., and Ajabor, L. (1972). J. Clin. Endocrinol. Metab. 34, 671-675.
Zarrow, M. X. and Gallo, R. V. (1969). Action of progesterone on PMS-induced ovulation in the immature rat. Endocrinology 84, 1274-1276.
Zeilmaker, G. H. (1966). The biphasic effect of progesterone on ovulation in the rat. Acta Endocrinol. (Copenhagen) 51, 461-468.

DISCUSSION AFTER DR. GORSKI'S PAPER

Dr. Jackson

I'd like to talk briefly about the relationship between the nervous system and hormonal control of the preovulatory surge of LH in one other species, namely the ewe. In the first study, the question asked was does the ewe have a circadian clock controlling the timing of the preovulatory LH surge? In other words, does she have a critical period?

If one injects estrogen into the anestrous ewe, there occurs approximately 12 hours later a surge of LH which approximates the preovulatory surge of LH. At least it is a similar type of response. Injection of estrogen into the female rat can also induce release of LH. However, the LH surge will occur only in the afternoon, regardless of when estrogen is given, due to the presence of a neural clock. I reasoned that if there was no critical period or clock in the ewe, an injection of estrogen would cause the LH surge to occur at a constant interval following the time at which the estrogen was injected rather than at a specific hour of day. Fifty micrograms of estradiol were injected into anestrous ewes either at six in the morning, at noon, or at six in the evening, and then blood samples were taken every three hours for 27 hours. An LH peak means a change from a base-line level of two or three nanograms per milliliter up to approximately 250 nanograms per milliliter. Table 1 shows that the interval at which the peak occurred was essentially

TABLE 1. TIME OF LH RELEASE AND INTERVAL BETWEEN INJECTION OF ESTRADIOL BENZOATE AND ELEVATION OF SERUM LH LEVELS IN ANESTROUS EWES.

Group	Hour of Injection	Interval to LH Peak (hr)[a]	Time of LH Peak[a]
A	0600	13.3 ± 0.73	1920 ± 0.73 hr[b]
B	1200	12.6 ± 0.60	0036 ± 0.60 hr[b]
C	1800	12.0 ± 2.24	0600 ± 2.24 hr[b]
D[c]	0630	No Elevation of LH Levels	

[a] *Mean ± SEM.*

[b] *Significantly different from each other ($P < 0.01$).*

[c] *Group D received oil.*

constant following the time of the injection, and that peaks occurred at several hours of the day. This suggests that the ewe does not have a circadian clock controlling the timing of the estrogen-induced release of LH.

Figure 1 compares the type of system known to occur in the rat with that postulated for the ewe. In the rats, the LH surge occurs when the daily change in neural sensitivity coincides with the presence of estrogen. In the ewe there is no daily change in neural sensitivity, and it is the rising estrogen levels which are primarily responsible for timing the preovulatory LH surge. Studies reported by Knobil's group suggest that the monkey may also have the "type two" system (Figure 1).

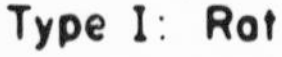

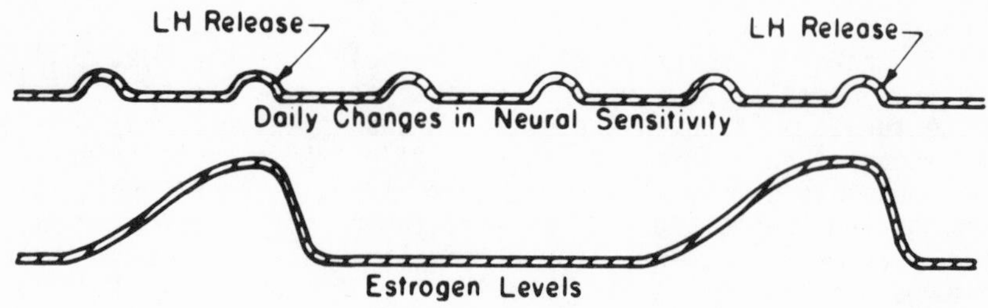

Type II: Ewe

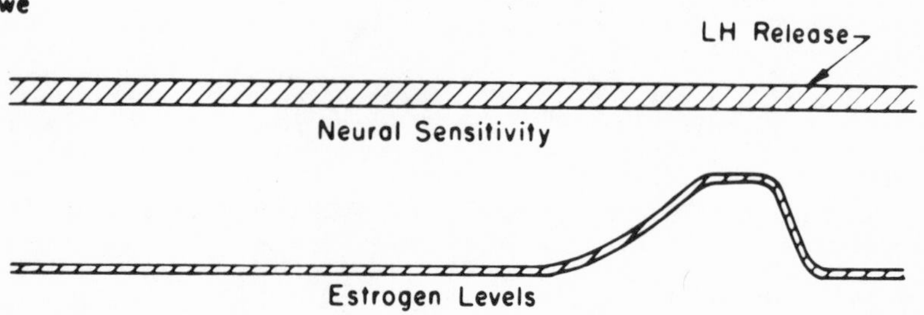

Figure 1. Two basic types of interaction between neural centers and estrogen leading to the preovulatory surge of LH.

Dr. Ramaley

I have a comment on Dr. Gorski's paper. You mentioned the role of adrenal hormones in controlling the cycle and I have plenty of data, and so do a lot of people, that rather subtle phase shifts in either corticosterone or maybe progesterone can influence the cycle. For example, if you shift the phase of the adrenal rhythm in developing mice, you suppress fertility; while in the adult, you seem to enhance fertility. I think this is an area of considerable interest. In this symposium, we haven't covered the maturing animal in which probably there's a need for synchronizing these hundreds of rhythms we're beginning to point out. And it's very likely that an animal can synchronize itself with any of a variety of these rhythms. I've emphasized the adrenal. Russ Reiter has emphasized the pineal, and you are interested in neural rhythms. But we should keep in mind in this conference that subtle phase shifts amongst these are very important and each of us is concerned with one or another.

Dr. Gorski

I think that is certainly a good point. Although we think in terms of a 24-hour clock for ovulation in the rat, as I indicated, progesterone has been shown to advance ovulation by three or four hours. Again, a very small phase shift, but one which could be very important. This concept of many rhythms coinciding, or synchronizing into a particularly important rhythm, at least for our scientific interests, does include the possibility of significant phase shifts. Earlier we saw what happens, at least mathematically, when various rhythms get in and out of phase. Physiologically, something important happens as well.

Dr. Karsch

Along the lines of clarification, I did not mean to indicate that gonadal steroids have no effect on pituitary responsiveness to synthetic LRF in the monkey. Certainly they do, at least under experimental circumstances. The important point is this; thus far we have not been able to reach the physiological significance of our findings. These experiments are described in detail elsewhere (Krey et al., 1973) and I will discuss only a few of the salient features here. To examine whether estradiol enhances pituitary responsiveness to releasing factor, we administered fixed doses of LRF to Rhesus monkeys at various stages of the menstrual cycle when circulating estradiol levels are changing. The resultant increases in circulating LH were largest when releasing factor was administered during the preovulatory LH surge, a stage when circulating estradiol levels are maximal. During the late follicular phase, however, when circulating estradiol is also quite high, the response was smallest, notably less than during the early follicular or luteal phases when serum estradiol levels are relatively low. Thus, we were unable to conclude from these experiments that estradiol enhanced the response of the monkey pituitary to LRF. It should be emphasized, however, that estradiol is only one of many hormonal variables during the menstrual cycle and we next utilized ovariectomized monkeys so that we could manipulate circulating estradiol as the only steroidal variable.

Much to our surprise we observed that in the ovariectomized monkey, physiological increments in circulating estradiol diminished the magnitude of the response to a fixed dose of LRF. Curiously, the duration of these diminished responses was prolonged. If any conclusion is warranted from these studies, it must be that in the physiological setting of the menstrual cycle of the monkey, the importance of gonadal steroids in modulating pituitary responsiveness to LRF must still be determined.

The second point I would like to make concerns the possible role of progesterone in triggering the LH surge. As you indicated, adrenal progesterone probably plays an important role in the rat; there is some compelling evidence for this view. We have considered this possibility for the primate and have reached the conclusion that progesterone, either adrenal or ovarian, plays little or no role in the induction of the LH surge. This is based on three lines of evidence. First, in our estrogen suppressed ovariectomized females, we can induce an LH surge, which closely resembles the preovulatory LH discharge of intact monkeys, without any measurable change in circulating progesterone levels. Secondly, LH surges can be induced in ovariectomized-adrenalectomized monkeys by the administration of estrogen. Thirdly, neither the spontaneous nor the estrogen-induced LH surge in the monkey is coupled to the time of day, thus suggesting that circadian adrenal rhythms do not play a role in the LH surge mechanism.

Dr. Gorski

First let me say the obvious, that the rat isn't a monkey or human and vice-versa. You said that you don't think adrenal progesterone is necessary for ovulation in the monkey. However, if we look at the broad picture, what is necessary and what happens can be two different things. If following anterior deafferentation of the preoptic area, rats can ovulate, perhaps none of the rest of the brain is necessary for ovulation in the rat. Yet, I'm sure it is involved. In the case of ovarian feedback you have very clearly shown a role for estrogen in the monkey where you can actually measure blood levels after treatment. In the rat, hormone levels are just beginning to be measured so there is much speculation. But taking the primate work, it is very clear that estrogen alone can trigger the LH surge. But progesterone could also participate. I think there are many modulating factors, and in some way, some part of the brain or maybe the pituitary -- something has to decide what the appropriate response is. So my own philosophy is first, to find out what is actually essential and then to identify these modulating factors. I agree with your experimental approach; I think we ought to keep in mind though, that which we rule out as non-essential may play a role.

Your data on the responsiveness of the pituitary are very interesting and remind me of the recent paper by Schally, et al. (1973). In this study they were interested in the problem of explaining differences in the release of FSH and LH following the administration of a single releasing factor. They studied pituitary response in vitro and as you have just reported, they see a complex dose dependent effect; at one level of steroid LH increases but FSH doesn't, at another level of steroid FSH release increases while LH goes down. It is clear that the influence of hormones directly at the pituitary is very complicated. In one sense, we owe this important question to Bogdanove who kept us honest. While many of us jumped on the bandwagon that neuroendocrine regulation took place at the level of the brain, Bogdanove suggested that perhaps there was regulation at the pituitary as well. It now appears that important regulation takes place at both levels.

Dr. Halberg

Dr. Gorski made the point that I wanted to make and that is, what can we conclude from, say step-wise ablations of the brain or from, say hypothalamic or pituitary island or from studies in vitro, say in organ culture. I would like to point out, with respect to your fine presentation, that Dr. R. Andrews of Nebraska and Ronald hiotsuka by culturing, in our laboratory, hamster adrenals in vitro, have been able to find a rhythm in corticosterone production in the absence of ACTH. These are adrenals that are cultured for several days, in organ culture, presumably under constant conditions. None of us would be so foolhardy to conclude that we all, as intact human beings, do everything we do just on the basis of an endogenous rhythm.

The adrenal rhythm "generator" responds to ACTH, of course. My suggestion and question to you and to others would be this: In studying a spectrum of reproductive rhythms, could one do first, step-wise ablations and then switch to cultures of the pituitary and of the ovary, just as one cultures the adrenal? If we had a culture and we found, say ultradian or any other rhythms, one could see how these correspond in the end organ, the ovary and in the pituitary and the hypothalamus.

Dr. Gorski

Yes, ovarian cultures are being studied but from the point of view of the mechanism of gonadotrophin or HCG action on ovarian tissue.

Dr. Halberg

Several cycles for how many days?

Dr. Gorski

These investigators are looking at receptors within ovarian tissue, hormone receptors, so they haven't undertaken that type of chronological study, so far as I know.

Dr. Halberg

Does Dr. Karsch know about ovarian organ culture?

Dr. Karsch

Ovarian tissues have been cultured.

Dr. Halberg

For how long?

Dr. Karsch

Dr. Channing has cultured granulosa cells for several weeks, but to my knowledge she has not looked for rhythms.

Dr. Halberg

Did this involve the ovary or parts of it, or merely tissue culture?

Dr. Karsch

No, not the ovary in total.

Dr. Halberg

If somebody is sufficiently ambitious and really cultures an ovary, they should take it from a hibernator. We at Minnesota had picked the rat and mouse while Dr. Andrews (Nebraska) picked the hamster and succeeded; the hibernator's glands are apparently much better to culture.

Dr. Karsch

I have one more comment regarding the rapid rhythm in circulating LH observed in the ovariectomized monkey. It is something which is very intriguing and very mystifying at the same time. The results of Ferin, at Columbia, suggest that perhaps this rhythm originates in the pituitary, in that the rhythm persists when the pituitary gland is disconnected from the hypothalamus. Further, he observed a pulsatile rhythm when synthetic LH-releasing hormone is infused continuously. One of the characteristics of the circhoral rhythm in ovariectomized monkeys is that the rise in circulating LH during an oscillation always occurs within a 15-minute sampling period; and then the decline occurs over a longer period of approximately 1 hour. If the rhythm originates in the pituitary itself, this raises an intriguing question concerning how LH secreting cells in one portion of the pituitary are coordinated with LH secreting cells in another portion of the gland such that they secrete LH at the same time, or very near to the same time.

Dr. Gorski

It is intriguing. Just to throw out some speculation, maybe each cell puts out LH for only a minute. With a very short period of actual secretion, the degree of synchrony may be much less than that indicated by plasma LH. For another speculation, consider the fact that after castration there's a marked increase in numbers of LH producing cells. Where do these cells come from; perhaps from resting chromophobes? Can we think in terms of the cell cycle? Without proposing cell division, could we invoke changing cell cycles or some very important process so that each of these functionally new cells, so-to-speak, is exposed to LRF at the same time, and that this entrains a rhythm? You can see that I'm speculating.

My own prejudice, without personal experience, is that this rhythm, at least in the rat, is an expression of the secretory process in the pituitary under these conditions of very high, rapid activity. I was very interested when you mentioned the work on the primate. We know from the work of Malvin's laboratory at Purdue that there is an increase in cranial secretion, so episodic fluctuations are not a reflection of peripheral metabolism. But the cranium includes both the pituitary and the brain; is there a similar episodic rhythm in LRF secretion? My prejudice, as I say, right now is related to the very high activity of these cells, either neural or hypophyseal. Maybe under this condition, when they're really constantly working, somehow they become synchronized within the limits that we see. In any case, I agree it's a very interesting problem.

Dr. Prahlad

In many of these organ culture systems, serum is used. How do they take care of trophic hormones in serum?

Dr. Halberg

As best I know, serum is used by neither R. Andrews nor R. Shiotsuka. Otherwise, you have to live with the initial conditions, but you do not modify them later beyond replenishing mediums. In keeping with Dr. Reiter's suggestion, we shall look at the constancy of lighting.

Dr. Krieger

I just want to ask for information relating to the constancy of the tissue culture environment. In those experiments is the medium changed, and is it sampled periodically? Do you have a problem of pile-up of metabolic products of the hormone which you would not have, say if superfusion were performed?

Dr. Halberg

It is different from superfusion. As best we know, when the medium, a Trowell medium T8, is changed the replacement should be identical on each occasion. We try not to add or to subtract. Since you bring it up, however, the first studies done on rhythms in tissue culture were feeding phenomena because they replenished the medium and never controlled that factor.

DISCUSSION REFERENCES

Krey, L., Butler, W., Weiss, G., Weick, R., Dierschke, D., and Knobil, E. (1973). In: *Hypothalamic Hypophysiotropic Hormones* (Gual, C. and Rosenberg, E., eds.), pp. 39-47, Excerpta Medica, Amsterdam.

Schally, A. V., Redding, T. W., and Armmura, A. (1973). Endocrinology 93, 893-902.

EFFECTS OF VARIOUS HORMONES ON THE PITUITARY-ADRENAL AXIS

Julian I. Kitay

Division of Endocrinology and Metabolism
Departments of Internal Medicine and Physiology
School of Medicine
University of Virginia
Charlottesville, Virginia

Most discussions of the mechanisms concerned with regulation of the pituitary-adrenal axis consider only components intrinsic to the system. Current understanding of the essential factors involved may be summarized briefly as follows. Stimulatory and inhibitory inputs from a variety of sources converge on centers in the basal hypothalamus. These signals result in stimulation (or inhibition) of corticotropin releasing factor (CRF) secretion from the median eminence. CRF is transported via the hypothalamico-hypophyseal portal system to the anterior pituitary gland and stimulates adrenocorticotrophic hormone (ACTH) secretion; ACTH in turn, stimulates adrenal corticosteroid secretion. Corticosterone, the principle glucocorticoid hormone in the rat, is bound in plasma to corticosterone binding globulin (CBG); however, a fraction remains unbound in equilibrium with the bound portion. The liver clears circulating corticosteroids and metabolizes them, by reduction and conjugation, to inactive compounds which are excreted. Control of the axis is manifested at various levels: a) It responds to stressful inputs in an essentially open-loop fashion with an increase in adrenal steroid output; b) Otherwise, circulating steroid exerts negative feedback at the hypothalamus or the pituitary, or both; c) The liver participates by regulating steroid clearance rate; d) The regulatory role of CBG remains unclear; e) Circulating ACTH levels may also participate in short-loop negative feedback; f) The hypothalamic (?) circadian rhythm center modulates the CRF-ACTH-steroid sequence on a diurnal basis; and g) The homeostatic regulatory role of the central nervous system (CNS) centers is still uncertain.

Recent studies have demonstrated that hormones other than CRF, ACTH, and corticosterone may play significant roles in regulation of the pituitary-adrenal axis. These include testosterone, estradiol, prolactin, growth hormone, thyroxine, and melatonin. Evidence is available indicating that they affect pituitary ACTH secretion, adrenal steroido-

These studies were supported in part by a USPHS Research Grant (AM03370) from the NIH.

genesis, and/or peripheral steroid clearance in the rat, and to a lesser extent, in the hamster and mouse. Evaluation of the physiologic importance of these hormonal effects on adrenal function is complex. A major problem is that no single parameter provides a comprehensive assessment of the status of the system. The components, i.e., brain, pituitary, adrenal, liver, etc., clearly interact; moreover, some hormones affect more than one component simultaneously. The overall effect may be unidirectional and reinforcing, such as is the case with estradiol, or it may be variable and at least partially self-cancelling, as is the case with testosterone. Furthermore, individual hormones not only act directly at one or more sites (which themselves interact), but also several hormones may interact at the same site or one may mediate the actions of another. Examples of these complexities are provided by the results of a number of studies.

Estradiol stimulates pituitary ACTH secretion after stress (Coyne and Kitay, 1969). Hypothalamic CRF content is unaltered, but pituitary responsiveness to CRF _in vitro_ is enhanced. Adrenal corticosterone production is increased by estradiol both in the presence and absence of the pituitary gland (Kitay, Coyne, Newsom, and Nelson, 1965). However, the effect is observed in hypophysectomized rats only when ACTH replacement and estradiol are administered simultaneously. Estradiol increases binding of corticosterone to CBG in rat plasma (Gala and Westphal, 1965). Paradoxically, however, this is associated with a shortened biological half-time ($T_{1/2}$) (Kitay, 1963) in contrast to the prolongation seen in human subjects. Hepatic metabolism of corticosterone, chiefly A-ring reduction, is stimulated by estradiol (Kitay, 1963), but this effect requires the presence of the pituitary gland and involves a hormone other than ACTH (Colby, Gaskin, and Kitay, 1972).

Testosterone inhibits pituitary ACTH secretion in male rats _in vivo_ and decreases pituitary responsiveness to CRF _in vitro_ (Coyne and Kitay, 1971). These effects are opposite to those observed in female rats. Although adrenal weight is diminished by testosterone, presumably reflecting less ACTH release, both adrenal corticosterone output and adrenal responsiveness to ACTH are enhanced. The latter are also observed in hypophysectomized male rats and do not require replacement with ACTH (Kitay, Coyne, Nelson, and Newsom, 1966). Testosterone decreases CBG binding of corticosterone in plasma (Gala and Westphal, 1965) but also retards its clearance ($T_{1/2}$) from the circulation (Kitay, 1963). Hepatic A-ring reduction of corticosterone is diminished simultaneously through the intermediary of a pituitary hormone (Colby, Gaskin, and Kitay, 1972). Side-chain metabolism of corticosterone by the liver is inconsequential and is affected minimally, if at all, by testosterone. Different results are obtained when cortisol is used as substrate, but this steroid is heterologous to the rat (Colby and Kitay, 1972a).

More detailed study of the effects of gonadectomy and gonadal hormone replacement in the rat has provided evidence _in vitro_ for an intra-adrenal pathway for the biosynthesis of reduced metabolites of corticosterone such as 5 α-dihydrocorticosterone (DHB) and 3 β, 5 α-tetrahydrocorticosterone (THB) (Kitay, Coyne, and Swygert, 1970). Production of such compounds by adrenal tissue from intact rats is small compared to corticosterone output. Gonadectomy in either sex results in enhanced adrenal capacity to produce DHB and THB, i.e., increased 5 α-reductase activity, associated with a corresponding diminution in corticosterone output. Appropriate replacement with estradiol or testosterone reverses these effects of gonadectomy. Hypophysectomy likewise is followed by stimulation of adrenal 5 α-reductase activity but the response is more rapid -- within 24 hours or less compared to an interval of two weeks or more after gonadectomy (Kitay, Coyne, and Swygert, 1971). ACTH replacement reverses the effect of hypophysectomy.

As already noted, the data indicating intra-adrenal steroid reduction were obtained using adrenal tissue incubated in vitro. Observations in vivo were limited to indirect chemical measurements consistent with enhanced secretion of A-ring reduced metabolites by castrates (Kitay, Coyne, Swygert, and Gaines, 1971). Double-label isotope dilution studies indicated that THB was secreted in vivo, but the necessity for pooling plasma samples to obtain sufficient material for analysis precluded definitive statistical validation of the effects of gonadectomy. Colby and Kitay (1972b) thereupon employed the technique of competitive protein binding (CPB) (Murphy, 1967) to obtain quantitative evidence concerning effects of both testosterone and estradiol on DHB and THB secretion.

Treatment groups consisted of intact and castrate male and female rats and castrates replaced with the appropriate gonadal hormone. Adrenal vein blood was collected under pentobarbital anesthesia, and plasma extracts were chromatographed. Zones corresponding to those of authentic corticosterone, DHB and THB, were eluted and quantitated by CPB. The identity of DHB was validated by mass spectrometry, that of corticosterone and THB having been previously substantiated by infrared spectrometry (Kitay, Coyne, and Swygert, 1970). Corticosterone secretion was reduced (and adrenal 5 α-reductase was increased as previously noted) following removal of the testes. The decline in corticosterone was accompanied by four-fold increases or more in the secretion of DHB and THB. Enhanced production of these compounds fully accounted for the fall in corticosterone output. Thus, total steroid secretion was unaffected. Each of the effects of castration was reversed by replacement with testosterone. Following ovariectomy, corticosterone secretion fell to less than half the rate obtained in intact control female rats. As in the male, secretion of DHB and THB was significantly increased -- 3.2- and 2-fold, respectively. Total steroid secretion was significantly reduced by gonadectomy. All the effects of ovarian removal were prevented by estradiol replacement.

These data substantiate the role of adrenal 5 α-reductase as a site at which the gonadal hormones influence the composition of adrenocortical secretory products. In view of the comparable inhibitory effect of ACTH replacement on adrenal reductase activity in hypophysectomized rats, it also seemed of interest to evaluate this aspect of ACTH action in vivo (Colby, Caffrey, and Kitay, 1972). One week after hypophysectomy, corticosterone output in adrenal venous effluent of female rats fell to a minimal level ($< 1\%$ of control). Secretion of DHB and THB was also diminished. However, after hypophysectomy, A-ring reduced compounds comprised over 75% of the total steroid output measured, compared to less than 15% in the controls. Adrenal 5 α-reductase activity in vitro rose simultaneously to high levels as expected. Administration of a single dose of ACTH to hypophysectomized rats 10 minutes prior to collection of adrenal venous effluent did not affect reductase activity. Steroid output rose somewhat but the predominance of reduced metabolites was unaltered. ACTH replacement for 1 to 2 days resulted in relatively slight changes in this pattern. After three days, reductase activity declined concomitant with a proportionately greater increase in corticosterone than DHB and THB output; however, the latter two compounds still predominated. Only after seven days of ACTH replacement did corticosterone output clearly exceed that of the two reduced metabolites combined, and this was associated with a further diminution in adrenal reductase activity in vitro. However, neither the pattern of steroid secretion nor reductase activity were restored to control levels at this time.

The reduced capacity of the adrenal to produce and secrete corticosteroids after hypophysectomy can be attributed, for the most part, to atrophic changes in the various processes essential to steroidogenesis, especially utilization of cholesterol. However, the preceeding observations indicate that the changes in steroid secretion following hypophysectomy are qualitative as well as quantitative. Production of reduced metabolites were observed to exceed that of corticosterone per se, a pattern which persisted until ACTH replacement resulted in a substantial lowering of adrenal 5 α-reductase activity. The extent to which 5 α-reduction may serve as a mechanism for physiologic regulation of adrenal steroid release in intact rats is unclear. The data demonstrate that changes in reductase activity in vitro clearly correlate with alterations in the profile of steroid secretion in vivo. Both the sex hormones and ACTH affect adrenal function through this mechanism. In other organs, 5 α-reduction is associated with the formation of biologically active steroids (Bruchovsky and Wilson, 1968). However, DHB and THB are generally thought to be inactive metabolites of corticosterone. These adrenal products are structurally identical to those normally obtained after incubation of corticosterone with hepatic tissue and are associated with the processes of clearance and excretion. The biological significance of increased adrenal secretion of such reduced compounds in response to gonadectomy or hypophysectomy remains to be established.

Detailed studies of the properties of the adrenal 5 α-reductase were then undertaken: a) to characterize the enzyme more adequately; b) to analyze the nature of the changes in its activity after gonadectomy and hypophysectomy; and c) to delineate the mechanisms involved in its control at the cellular level (Caffrey and Kitay, 1973). Four treatment groups, intact, orchiectomized, ovariectomized, and hypophysectomized, were used as tissue donors. Reductase activity was shown to reside almost exclusively in the microsomal fraction in each case. Activity is insensitive to hydrogen ion concentration between pH 6.0 and 7.5 but diminishes sharply outside this range. The enzyme is also insensitive to changes in ionic strength. The apparent K_m with respect to corticosterone is 4.5×10^{-5} M. Each of these characteristics is essentially the same regardless of treatment of the animal donors. There is measurable enzyme activity using a number of different Δ4,3-keto steroids including cortisol, 11-deoxycorticosterone (DOC), 11-deoxycortisol, testosterone, and androstenedione, as well as corticosterone. Mixing experiments were performed to evaluate the presence of an enzyme inhibitor or activator. When adrenal tissue from high and low enzyme activity states were mixed and incubated, the resultant rate observed was not different from that expected from the incubation of the tissues separately, suggesting the absence of a dissociable activator or inhibitor. There were, however, significant differences among the enzyme rates observed with different substrates. Androstenedione, testosterone, and DOC were metabolized most rapidly, whereas cortisol was metabolized most slowly. However, no differences in substrate preference were observed upon comparison of results with enzyme from each of the four sources. The temporal appearance of enzyme activity following hypophysectomy was studied for four weeks. It was found to increase steadily for two weeks (0.85 $\pm$ 0.62 to 84.0 $\pm$ 5.0 μg, corticosterone reduced per 10 mg/hour). Increases were evident in both enzyme concentration and total enzyme content per adrenal gland. Concentration remained high throughout, whereas content declined associated with progressive adrenal atrophy. Prior ovariectomy had no effect on the rate of enzyme appearance post-hypophysectomy. Likewise, estradiol replacement shortly after gland excision did not affect enzyme activity as measured 12 hours later. ACTH and testosterone did halt the enzyme activity rise compared to controls at a level which would be expected to have existed at the time of injection. The protein synthesis inhibitor, cycloheximide, also blocked the rise after hypophysectomy in a temporal pattern identical to that of ACTH and testosterone. Immediate corticosterone replacement in hypophysectomized animals was without significant effect on enzyme activity. The data suggest that the enzyme from each of the four treatment sources is identical and that the post-operative rise in activity reflects increased synthesis of enzyme due to removal of hormonal inhibition of specific protein synthetic mechanisms.

The initial studies demonstrating increased adrenal 5 α-reductase activity after gonadectomy were limited to enzyme assays using mature rats, gonadectomized either pre- or post-pubertally as donors. More detailed investigation revealed that the emergence of 5 α-reductase activity in response to gonadectomy is, at least in part, a maturational phenomenon (Witorsch and Kitay, 1972a). Castration of adult rats produces a deficit in corticosterone production and increased reductive capacity within two weeks. In rats gonadectomized during the third week of life, the deficit in adrenal corticosterone production is not seen until approximately seven weeks of age, which corresponds to the time when adrenal reductase activity is first demonstrable. The possibility that this observation is related to the duration of gonadal deficiency and not chronological age *per se*, was examined by measuring reductase activity 4, 6, and 9 weeks after neonatal gonadectomy. Duration seems unimportant, since, under such circumstances, reductase was not demonstrable 4 or 6 weeks post-operation but did appear after the normal age of puberty. In contrast, reductase activity increased promptly (within 24 hours) after hypophysectomy at 28 days of age. Thus, the capacity for A-ring reduction exists prior to puberty and is apparently under inhibitory control by the pituitary gland.

The effects of individual pituitary hormones on adrenal 5 α-reductase activity were evaluated in another series of experiments (Witorsch and Kitay, 1972b). Administration of FSH, LH, or TSH to hypophysectomized rats did not modify the high reductase levels obtained in saline-treated controls. In contrast, injection of ACTH, prolactin (0.5 mg/day), or growth hormone (1.0 mg/day) significantly lowered reductase activity. The inhibitory response to ACTH was expected (Kitay, Coyne, and Swygert, 1971). The parallel effects of prolactin and growth hormone are of interest since overlapping actions of the two have been noted frequently (Apostolakis, 1968). Of the several pituitary hormones observed to lower reductase activity in hypophysectomized rats, only prolactin was also inhibitory when administered to ovariectomized animals. The minimal dose of prolactin required was about 10 μg/day -- comparable to those required to produce luteotropic (Ahmad, Lyons, and Ellis, 1969) and mammotropic (Kumaresan, Anderson, and Turner, 1966) effects.

Most recently, the role of the pineal gland in regulating adrenal function has been evaluated in preliminary experiments (Ogle and Kitay, 1974). Female rats were either pinealectomized or sham-operated at 24 days of age. As expected, adrenal 5 α-reductase levels were high and corticosterone production low at six and eight weeks of age as a result of ovariectomy (Table 1). Pinealectomy minimized both effects at six weeks but not eight weeks. In another study melatonin was administered to intact female rats at a dose of 50 μg twice daily for seven days.

TABLE 1. EFFECTS OF PINEALECTOMY ON ADRENAL FUNCTION IN OVARIECTOMIZED RATS.

Treatment	Corticosterone Production[a]		Adrenal 5 α-Reductase Activity[a]	
	6 weeks	8 weeks	6 weeks	8 weeks
Sham-operated	1.0 ± 0.1	0.6 ± 0.1	6.4 ± 1.4	19.3 ± 0.9
Pinealectomized	1.5 ± 0.1*	0.8 ± 0.2	0.8 ± 0.9*	16.1 ± 3.2

[a] *Expressed as μg corticosterone/10 mg adrenal wt/hr.*

* *$P < 0.01$*

N = 6 to 12/group.

Secretion rate of DHB + THB in adrenal venous blood was increased 3-fold while that of corticosterone remained unchanged (Table 2). Finally, administration of melatonin to pinealectomized, hypophysectomized rats resulted in a significant increment in adrenal 5 α-reductase activity, above that produced by hypophysectomy alone (Table 3).

TABLE 2. EFFECTS OF MELATONIN ON ADRENAL STEROID OUTPUT IN INTACT FEMALE RATS.

Steroid	Saline	Melatonin
Adrenal Vein:		
Corticosterone (μg/hr)	31.5 ± 2.0	39.5 ± 4.2
DHB + THB (μg/hr)	8.1 ± 1.1	24.3 ± 4.8*
Corticosterone:Total (%)	81.0 ± 2.0	58.0 ± 5.0*

$^{*}P < 0.01$

N = 9 or 10/group.

TABLE 3. EFFECTS OF MELATONIN ON ADRENAL 5 α-REDUCTASE ACTIVITY IN PINEALECTOMIZED-HYPOPHYSECTOMIZED RATS.

Treatment	N	Adrenal Reductase[a]
Saline	9	18.8 ± 2.3
Melatonin	12	26.1 ± 1.8*

[a] *Expressed as μg corticosterone/10 mg adrenal wt/hr.*

$^{*}P < 0.02$

Conclusions concerning these observations must remain tentative. Melatonin is the only hormone tested to date which enhances the secretion of reduced metabolites by the adrenal gland. Its physiologic role, and indeed those of the pituitary hormones which are inhibitory, require further study both of their individual and their interactive effects.

REFERENCES

Ahmad, N., Lyons, W. R., and Ellis, S. (1969). Luteotrophic activity of rat hypophysial mammotrophin. Endocrinology 85, 378-380.

Apostolakis, M. (1968). Prolactin. Vitam. Horm. 26, 197-235.

Bruchovsky, N. and Wilson, J. D. (1968). The conversion of testosterone to 5 α-androstan-17 β-ol-3-one by rat prostate *in vivo* and *in vitro*. J. Biol. Chem. 243, 2012-2021.

Caffrey, J. L. and Kitay, J. I. (1973). Hormonal influences on the expression of adrenal 5 α-reductase. Fed. Proc. 32, 255.

Colby, H. D., Caffrey, J. L., and Kitay, J. I. (1972). Relation of adrenal 5 α-reductase activity to adrenocortical secretion *in vivo*. Excerpta Med. Found. Int. Congr. Ser., No. 256, 41.

Colby, H. D., Gaskin, J. H., and Kitay, J. I. (1972). Requirement of the pituitary gland for gonadal hormone effects on hepatic corticosteroid metabolism in rats and hamsters. Endocrinology 92, 769-774.

Colby, H. D. and Kitay, J. I. (1972a). Sex and substrate effects on hepatic corticosteroid metabolism. Endocrinology 90, 473-478.

Colby, H. D. and Kitay, J. I. (1972b). Effects of gonadal hormones on adrenocortical secretion of 5 α-reduced metabolites of corticosterone in the rat. Endocrinology 91, 1523-1527.

Coyne, M. D. and Kitay, J. I. (1969). Effect of ovariectomy on pituitary secretion of ACTH. Endocrinology 85, 1097-1102.

Coyne, M. D. and Kitay, J. I. (1971). Effect of orchiectomy on pituitary secretion of ACTH. Endocrinology 89, 1024-1028.

Gala, R. R. and Westphal, U. (1965). Corticosteroid-binding globulin in the rat. Studies on the sex difference. Endocrinology 77, 841-851.

Kitay, J. I. (1963). Pituitary-adrenal function in the rat after gonadectomy and gonadal hormone replacement. Endocrinology 73, 253-260.

Kitay, J. I., Coyne, M. D., Nelson, R., and Newsom, W. (1966). Relation of the testes to adrenal enzyme activity and adrenal corticosterone production in the rat. Endocrinology 78, 1061-1066.

Kitay, J. I., Coyne, M. D., Newsom, W., and Nelson, R. (1965). Relation of the ovary to adrenal corticosterone production and adrenal enzyme activity in the rat. Endocrinology 77, 902-908.

Kitay, J. I., Coyne, M. D., and Swygert, N. (1970). Influence of gonadectomy and replacement with estradiol or testosterone on formation of 5 α-reduced metabolites of corticosterone by the adrenal gland of the rat. Endocrinology 87, 1257-1265.

Kitay, J. I., Coyne, M. D., and Swygert, N. (1971). Effects of hypophysectomy and administration of cortisone or ACTH on adrenal 5 α-reductase activity and steroid production. Endocrinology 89, 432-438.

Kitay, J. I., Coyne, M. D., Swygert, N., and Gaines, K. E. (1971). Effects of gonadal hormones and ACTH on the nature and rates of secretion of adrenocortical steroids by the rat. Endocrinology 89, 565-570.

Kumaresan, P., Anderson, R. R., and Turner, C. W. (1966). Effect of graded levels of lactogenic hormone upon mammary gland growth and lactation in rats. Proc. Soc. Exp. Biol. Med. 123, 581-584.

Murphy, B. E. P. (1967). Some studies of the protein-binding of steroids and their application to the routine micro and ultramicro measurement of various steroids in body fluids by competitive protein-binding radioassay. J. Clin. Endocrinol. Metab. 27, 973-990.

Ogle, T. F. and Kitay, J. I. (1974). Pineal effects on adrenal steroidogenesis. Fed. Proc. 33, 287.

Witorsch, R. J. and Kitay, J. I. (1972a). Influence of the ovary, pituitary and age on adrenal 5 α-reductase activity in the rat. Endocrinology 90, 1374-1379.

Witorsch, R. J. and Kitay, J. I. (1972b). Pituitary hormones affecting adrenal 5 α-reductase activity: ACTH, growth hormone, and prolactin. Endocrinology 91, 764-769.

DISCUSSION AFTER DR. KITAY'S PAPER

Dr. Dellmann

When we look at experimental animals we usually measure only one parameter and your studies show very nicely that we certainly ought to take many more into consideration.

Dr. Craig

I was interested to note that you used TSH on this system. Have you ever tried thyroxine or, I should say, a lack of thyroxine, like thyroidectomized animals?

Dr. Kitay

That is an interesting question. Studies reported by Labrie and collaborators have suggested that the effects of estradiol on adrenal function are mediated through the thyroid gland. Using the variables I have discussed, we have been unable to demonstrate the intermediary of thyroid hormone with respect to the effects of either ACTH or the gonadal hormones. I hasten to say that there is considerable evidence relating the effects of thyroid hormone to corticosterone binding globulin. That is another matter altogether which raises a number of interesting questions because, as I indicated in passing, increased plasma protein-binding in the rat is associated with <u>accelerated</u> biological half-time.

Dr. Craig

The reason I asked this question is because, in recent work with thyroidectomized animals, a large drop in adrenal cortex content, plasma concentration, and secretion rates was noted. I was curious if you had performed similar studies, and if so, what the results were. We know that thyroxine is important, but we are not sure how it affects the adrenal; also we know that exercise and age seem to affect the adrenal. I wonder if you looked into this or have you even had time to think about it?

Dr. Kitay

If you mean direct effects of thyroxine on adrenal steroid output, I didn't mean to comment on that but rather only to the data I presented. I don't think there is an effect of thyroid hormone on adrenal reductase activity, at least we have not been able to demonstrate one directly. I support your observation that thyroidectomy leads to a diminution in steroid output. It also has other effects, as I have said, on binding and biological half-time and on other parameters, but not those that I discussed here.

Dr. Sellner

Do you know of any data relating either endogenous or exogenous prostaglandin concentrations to either reductase or steroid dehydrogenase?

Dr. Kitay

No.

Dr. Reiter

The effect of melatonin on alpha reductase was obviously independent of the pituitary since it occurred in hypophysectomized animals. The effects of pinealectomy could be explained, I believe, on the basis of an exaggerated ACTH secretion. Is that correct?

Dr. Kitay

Could be, yes.

Dr. Reiter

If that is true, your findings fit well with what we apparently know about the pineal gland and the ACTH secretion. After pinealectomy, there seems to be only a transitory stimulation of ACTH and this would explain, of course, the effect at six weeks and not later. So it isn't necessary to conclude that the effect of pinealectomy, which you reported, was aided by melatonin.

Dr. Kitay

At that point, no; that is why we went on to do more studies.

Dr. Reiter

I will say that melatonin generally seems to have effects on enzymes in the adrenals and in the testes. It seems that melatonin, and indeed the pineal gland, is becoming a little bit like one of Al Capp's characters in "Little Abner." He used to describe a character called a "Schmoo" which was anything you wanted it to be. Apparently the pineal and melatonin fall into this category. If you test them properly, they will have an effect somewhere on something virtually all the time.

Dr. Ramaley

I think we all look at those parts of your data that fit our interests, and I notice that you tried FSH or LH effects and didn't get anything. Now, in a lot of my studies I run across the finding that if I induce precocious puberty with PMS, I find changes in blood levels of corticosterone. I can get some of these same effects, although much diminished, in the ovariectomized animals, and I wonder if you have any comment. I would like to know at what level the PMS is acting. Have you ever tried PMS in your system?

Dr. Kitay

We have published data which relates to advancing the age of puberty. This was based on the assumption that puberty might be the signal which told the adrenal to make reduced compounds. Ray Witorsch, working in my laboratory, administered estrogen and progesterone in a cyclic fashion appropriate for the rat, for two or three cycles beginning around 21 days of age. Despite clear-cut effects on uterine and vaginal morphology, there were no changes in appearance of adrenal reductase activity after ovariectomy. We also administered FSH and LH, only to be complete, because neonatal gonadectomy undoubtedly resulted in elevated levels of endogenous gonadotrophins within a few days. However, even in the case of neonatally gonadectomized animals, achievement of the age normally associated with puberty was required to demonstrate an adrenal response.

Dr. Reiter

I just want to make one comment about melatonin. It could well be the pineal hormone that is important for many of the physiological functions we have examined. The other possibility is that the indoleamines within the pineal gland have something to do with the release of the true pineal hormone, e.g., a polypeptide. If this is true, I think that it would be wise for some of us, myself included, to test the effects of melatonin in pinealectomized animals.

Dr. Kitay

This is part of the reason that we did not think that melatonin was solely responsible for the effects. So we have no disagreement. Melatonin does not behave as it ought in pinealectomized-hypophysectomized rats; and this is why we are preparing other fractions from the pineal to look for what we think is probably a more relevant substance, a peptide specifically.

Dr. Franz

Do you have additional evidence that the increase in the reductase activity, e.g., after hypophysectomy, was due to an increased de novo synthesis of the enzyme other than the cycloheximide work? It would be possible that, for example, cycloheximide could be inhibiting a system which degrades the enzyme, thereby giving an increased steady-state level in that way. To exclude this you would have to use immunological methodology.

Dr. Kitay

We have not excluded the possibilities you suggest.

Dr. Halberg

In 1960, we reported (Halberg and Haus, 1960) that in two populations of mice (one inbred, the other hybrid), adrenal corticosterone levels determined at the time of peak physiologic secretion differed consistently within the two sexes. The female glands, heavier than those of males, had the higher content and concentration of corticosterone. It seems useful to carry out single sample comparisons at a defined circadian time.

Dr. Dellmann

After hypophysectomy, you found an increased DHB (5 α-dihydroxycorticosterone) and a decreased corticosterone, is that correct; and when you added ACTH you had the same relationship? Now, how long would it take, how many days or hours after administration of ACTH to reestablish the normal corticosterone and DHB values?

Dr. Kitay

It took almost two weeks under conditions we selected. I think the timing of results depends on both the amount of ACTH administered and the kind of ACTH. In the studies I presented, we used both ACTH gel and an experimental depot preparation much superior with respect to maintenance of blood levels and stimulation of the adrenal. There is no question in my mind that the predominant effect of ACTH is to stimulate steroid synthesis by accelerating the conversion of cholesterol to pregnenolone. Your question gives me the opportunity to reemphasize that point. I do not wish to minimize or refute the generally held view of the importance of ACTH to that aspect of steroid output. One sees an immediate response to ACTH in terms of total steroid production. In a sense, you might liken reductase activity to a faucet at the output end of the adrenal. ACTH also works at that site as well as working on steroid biosynthesis. The response at the input end is much more rapid, and one sees then a greater total steroid output promptly. The change in steroid composition begins to occur about three or four days after ACTH replacement. Precise estimates of timing are difficult because what we are looking at is adrenal repair. The animals have been hypophysectomized for one week and have adrenal atrophy so that the process involves repair rather than maintenance.

DISCUSSION REFERENCES

Halberg, F. and Haus, E. (1960). Am. J. Physiol. 199, 859-862.

CIRCADIAN PITUITARY ADRENAL RHYTHMS

Dorothy T. Krieger

Division of Endocrinology
Department of Medicine
Mount Sinai School of Medicine
New York City, New York 10029

INTRODUCTION

A circadian periodicity of plasma corticosteroid levels has been well established in many species, including the human (Migeon, Tyler, Mahoney, Florentin, Castle, Bliss and Samuels, 1956; Halberg, 1969; Dusseau and Meier, 1971; Singley and Chavin, 1971). The present report will attempt to define the characteristics of such periodicity and describe experimental approaches, both in animals and humans, which have been designed to delineate the factors underlying this periodicity.

Plasma corticosteroid levels normally peak in the period preceding the onset of awakening or activity, with a progressive decline over the ensuing twenty-four hour period (Perkoff, Eik-Nes, Nugent, Fred, Nimer, Rush, Samuels and Tyler, 1959; Guillemin, Dear and Liebilt, 1959). Such periodicity is not posture-dependent (Vernikos-Danellis, Leach, Winget, Rambaut and Mack, 1971), is reproducible with regard to level and pattern (Krieger, Allen, Rizzo and Krieger, 1971) and in the human is apparently not altered by prolonged fasting (Marti, Studer, Dettweiler and Rohner, 1969) or short periods of continuous feeding (Krieger, Allen, Rizzo and Krieger, 1971). Hepatic dysfunction with resultant decreased cortisol removal may result in obliteration of periodicity (Tucci, Albacete and Martin, 1966). Reversal of the day/night schedule results in a phase reversal of the circadian pattern within a variable time interval (Perkoff, Eik-Nes, Nugent, Fred, Nimer, Rush, Samuels and Tyler, 1959). Initial animal and human studies delineating corticosteroid circadian periodicity were based on a sampling frequency of every 4 to 6 hours over the twenty-four hour period with the resultant curves obtained describing a smooth rise and fall over this time period. Subsequent studies in the human, based upon a sampling frequency of every 30 (Krieger, 1969; Krieger, Allen, Rizzo and Krieger, 1971) or 20 minutes (Hellman, Nakada, Curti, Weitzman, Kream, Roffward, Ellman, Fukushima and Gallagher, 1970), this frequency being chosen in view of the reported

---

Supported by Grant NB 0289397A2.

half-life of cortisol which varies between 60 and 90 minutes, have resulted in a more detailed description of the circadian pattern. It became apparent that episodic, relatively synchronous peaks of plasma adrenocorticotropic hormone (ACTH) and corticosteroid levels were evident throughout the day, with the majority of such peaks, however, still occurring in the period preceding the onset of awakening, with a

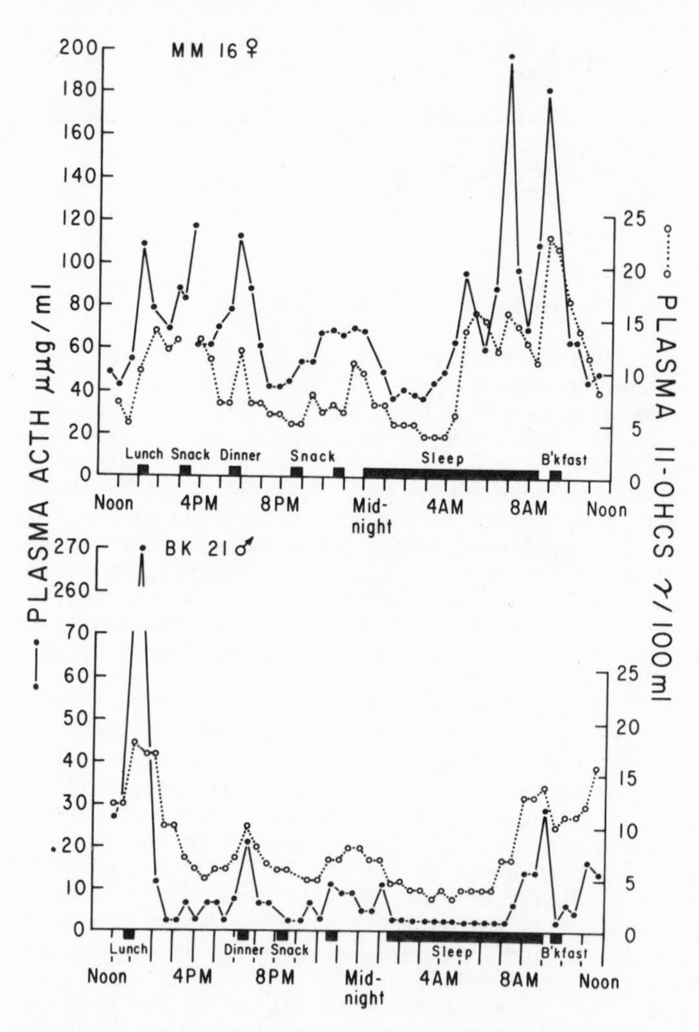

Figure 1. Circadian periodicity of plasma 11-hydroxycorticosteroid (11-OHCS) and plasma adrenocorticotropic hormone (ACTH) levels during a 24-hour period as determined by half-hourly sampling in two normal subjects. Meal time and sleep is indicated (Reproduced by permission, Krieger, Allen, Rizzo, and Krieger, 1971).

subsequent downward trend (Figure 1). We have suggested that this major rise of plasma corticosteroid and ACTH levels reflects circadian, neurally mediated release of corticotrophin-releasing factor (CRF), and consequently of ACTH, during a delimited "critical" period in the 24-hour cycle; with subsequent levels reflecting a combination of metabolic disposition and the effects of environmental or other endogenous stimuli on CRF release (Krieger and Krieger, 1967).

The question next arises as to the derivation of the source of such periodicity. The existence of such a circadian pattern cannot be explained by circadian alterations in the half-life or metabolic clearance of cortisol (DeLacerda, Kowarski and Migeon, 1973) or circadian variation in corticosteroid binding globulin concentrations (DeMoor, Heirwegh, Hermans and Declerck-Raskin, 1962). Although a circadian periodicity of adrenal corticoid release has been described in cultured hamster adrenal glands, the predominant factor regulating adrenal cortical secretion is ACTH. There are no data at present with regard to different half-lives of ACTH at different times of day. Evidence with regard to altered circadian adrenal responsiveness to ACTH is contradictory, evidence for this being present in the rat (Ungar, 1964) but not in the human (Nugent, Eik-Nes, Kent, Samuels and Tyler, 1960). Utilizing the frequent sampling techniques described above, it is evident that a correlation exists between peaks of plasma ACTH levels and those of plasma corticosteroids. Such ACTH periodicity is independent of feedback, since a circadian periodicity of plasma ACTH levels has also been reported in the human with Addison's disease (Graber, Givens, Nicholson, Island and Liddle, 1965; Besser, Orth, Nicholson, Byyny, Abe and Woodham, 1971) and in the adrenalectomized rat. These studies, however, cannot adequately define ACTH periodicity since the sampling time employed (twice daily in the human, and every four hours in the rat) greatly exceeds the reported half-life of ACTH, [8-25 minutes in the human (Besser, Cullen, Irvine, Ratcliffe and Landon, 1971) and 3-4 minutes in the rat (Matsuyama, Ruhmann-Wennhold, Johnson and Nelson, 1972)]. Since sampling every 5 minutes over the entire 24-hour cycle is not feasible in such Addisonian subjects, we have performed studies utilizing half-hourly sampling. It is apparent that these Addisonian subjects display the same pattern of episodic peaks superimposed over the circadian rise and fall of ACTH levels as is seen in normal subjects. Because of the lack of any steroid feedback in these subjects, however, the actual ACTH levels observed are much higher than those seen in normal individuals. Such a demonstration of ACTH periodicity in the absence of the adrenal gland is evidence both that the observed periodicity of plasma corticosteroid levels is a reflection of that of ACTH levels and that the periodicity of such ACTH levels is not merely a reflection of feedback processes.

Proceeding to a consideration as to the role of CRF involvement in the regulation of ACTH periodicity, there is no available evidence with regard to a circadian variation of pituitary responsiveness to CRF-like substances. Although bioassays for CRF are relatively insensitive, a circadian periodicity in the rat hypothalamic content of CRF has been reported (Hiroshige and Sakakura, 1971) which persists in hypophysectomized animals. Other evidence of neural involvement in the regulation of ACTH periodicity may be adduced from the finding that in both the rat and the human, a circadian periodicity of plasma corticosteroid levels is not present until the onset of what is equivalent to the age of the mid-prepubertal period (Franks, 1967; Allen and Kendall, 1967; Ader, 1969; Hiroshige and Sato, 1970). This is in contrast to the presence of normal adrenal responsiveness to ACTH (Jailer, 1950) and normal pituitary-adrenal stress responsiveness (Milkovic and Milkovic, 1966) well in advance of this age. In the rat, the age of appearance of periodicity of plasma corticosteroid levels also correlates with the time of appearance of periodicity of hypothalamic CRF levels (Takebe, Sakakura and Mashimo, 1972).

Since neurotransmitter regulation of circadian aspects of ACTH secretion is generally accepted (Krieger, 1973c) one would next look for evidence of periodicity in central nervous system (CNS) content of such transmitters. A CNS-regional periodicity of acetylcholine (Hanin, Massarelli and Costa, 1970), norepinephrine (Reis, Weinbren and Corvelli, 1968) and serotonin (Reis, Corvelli and Conners, 1969) has been observed in several animal species. Again, attainment of adult phase relationships of serotonin levels in the rat appears at approximately the same age as the appearance of adrenal circadian periodicity (Asano, 1971).

At this point one can next ask as to what the basis is for neural rhythmicity, be it that of neurotransmitter content, sleep-wake, or rest-activity cycles. One can ask if a given periodicity drives that of the other, whether one or all of these periodicities are secondary to a hormonal rhythm or whether each of these variables is affected independently by a given "pacemaker," perhaps light or light-dark transition. Numerous experimental protocols have been devised in an attempt to answer these questions. In the following sections a resumé of the pertinent findings of animal and human experiments will be cited and comparison made of the differences and similarities noted.

One approach has been to alter CNS content of the neurotransmitter agents known to affect ACTH release. It was reasoned that if there was a circadian periodicity of such CNS neurotransmitter content and if ACTH levels were responsive to changes in neurotransmitter concentrations, it should be possible to abolish the circadian rise in plasma corticosteroid levels by altering the CNS content of such transmitters within a period just prior to the time of the circadian rise. Obliteration of the circadian variation of plasma corticosteroid levels in the cat has been achieved by alteration of central neurotransmitter content or action; acetylcholine (Krieger, Silverberg, Rizzo and Krieger, 1968) and serotonin (Krieger and Rizzo, 1969) being effective in this regard. To date, it has not been possible to block the circadian rise of plasma corticosteroid levels in the human by the administration of either atropine or sodium phenobarbital. Likewise, administration in a therapeutic regimen over a two-week period of reserpine, chlordiazepoxide, meprobamate or chlorpromazine, or of diphenylhydantoin over a two- or eight-week period, has also been ineffective in blocking the circadian rise (Krieger and Krieger, 1967).

Another approach has been to evaluate the effect of discrete CNS lesions on corticosteroid periodicity. In the rat, anterior hypothalamic lesions (Slusher, 1964), complete hypothalamic deafferentiation

(Halász, Slusher and Gorski, 1967; Palka, Coyer and Critchlow, 1969; Greer, Panton and Allen, 1972), anterior hypothalamic deafferentiation (Moore and Eichler, 1972), fornix section (Moberg, Scapagnini, de Groot and Ganong, 1971; Lengvari and Halász, 1973), and suprachiasmatic lesions (Moore and Eichler, 1972) have been reported to obliterate corticosteroid periodicity. In the rat the effect of fornix section is only temporary (Lengvari and Halász, 1973). Section of the primary or accessory optic tracts in the rat (Moore and Eichler, 1972) does not affect corticosteroid periodicity. With the recent evidence of the existence of a retino-hypothalamic tract in the rat and hamster, and probably in primate species as well (Moore and Lenn, 1972), such a tract arising from the ganglion cells of the retina and terminating in the suprachiasmatic nuclei, it may well be that this tract has been severed by any of the procedures just cited as being effective in disrupting adrenal periodicity. It is also of interest that suprachiasmatic lesions have also been reported to abolish circadian drinking (cholinergically modulated) and activity patterns in the rat (Stephan and Zucker, 1972). Taken together, the foregoing observations, if confirmed, provide an anatomical basis to explain the interrelationship of light-modulated corticosteroid and motor (possible sleep) periodicity. Another point worthy of mention is that all lesions affecting periodicity in the rat essentially prevent the circadian rise rather than elevate trough corticosteroid levels. This would indicate that a stimulatory pathway had been severed and perhaps imply that, save for the period of the circadian rise and in association with ACTH stress induced output, inhibitory mechanisms are predominant over the remainder of the 24-hour cycle.

In the human, patients demonstrating disturbance of consciousness with either acute systemic disease (Sholiton, Werk and Marnell, 1961) or with chronic diffuse CNS disease (Perkoff, Eik-Nes, Nugent, Fred, Nimer, Rush, Samuels and Tyler, 1959) had been reported as showing absence or alteration of corticosteroid periodicity. These studies, however, gave no insight as to specific anatomical loci that might be involved. To date (Krieger, 1961; Krieger and Krieger, 1966; Krieger, 1973b) we have studied 43 conscious patients with radiographically and clinically localized hypothalamic or limbic system disease, of whom 53% had abnormal corticosteroid patterns. Rather than suppression of the circadian rise, this abnormality consisted of apparent phase reversal or occurrence of peaks of plasma corticosteroid levels at normally quiescent times of day. It is of interest that patients with Cushing's disease manifest the same type of irregular oscillations in plasma cortisol levels as seen in some of the patients with hypothalamic disease (Krieger, Allen, Rizzo and Kriger, 1971) (Figure 2). Such abnormality is present when the disease is clinically active or in remission. This finding, together with evidence of altered sleep EEG stages and lack of nocturnal growth hormone release in patients with both active disease and in remission, is suggestive of some central nervous dysfunction as being etiological in this disease (Krieger and Glick, 1972). In contrast, only 1 of 21 conscious patients with localized CNS disease outside the hypothalamic-limbic system area had an abnormal pattern. These studies would indicate that pathways involved in the regulation of circadian corticosteroid

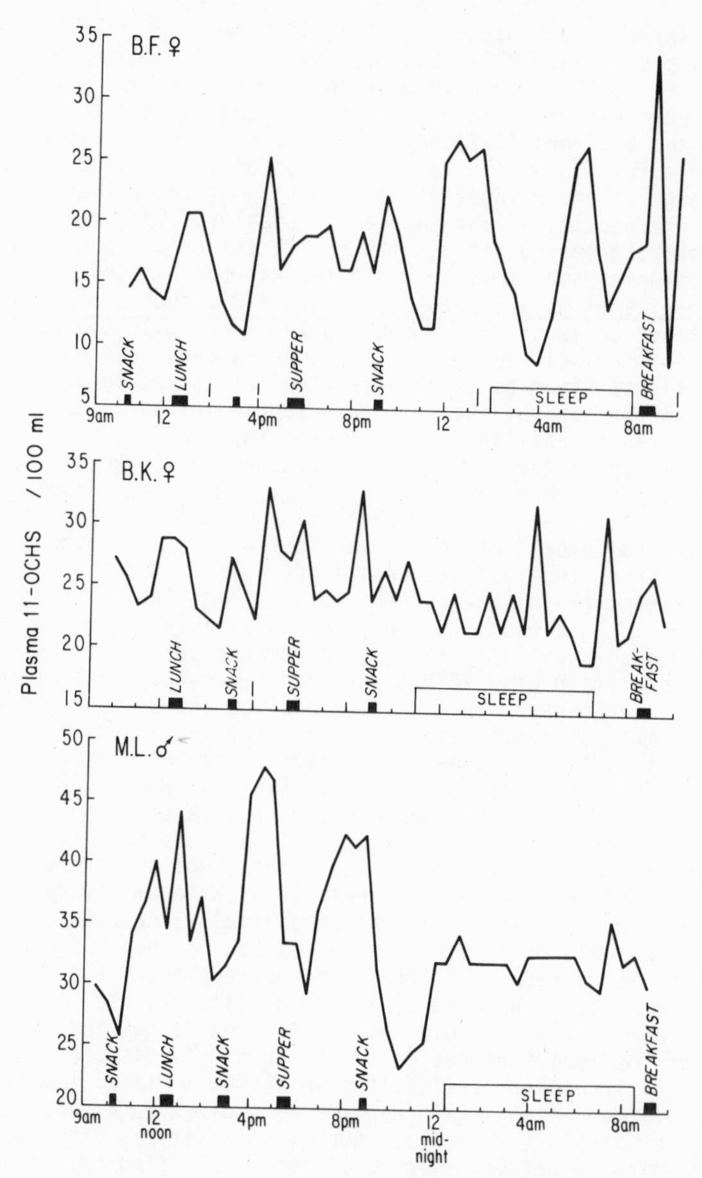

Figure 2. Circadian periodicity of plasma 11-hydroxycorticosteroid (11-OHCS) levels as determined by half-hourly sampling in three patients with Cushing's syndrome. Meal time and sleep are indicated. (Reproduced by permission, Krieger, Allen, Rizzo and Krieger, 1971).

periodicity in the human occupy a delimited CNS area, roughly similar to that demonstrated in animal lesion studies.

Patients with psychiatric disease may perhaps be considered as having "functional" CNS lesions. The circadian periodicity of corticosteroid levels has been most extensively studied in depressive states. There appears to be general agreement that such periodicity is normal, though maintained at higher plasma cortisol levels (Bridges and Jones, 1966; Fullerton, Wenzel, Lohrenz and Fahs, 1968; Carpenter and Bunney, 1971a) and is characterized by an increase in the number and duration of secretory episodes (Sachar, Hellman, Roffwarg, Halpern, Fukushima and Gallagher, 1973). A study of manic patients also reports normal periodicity , but there were only two sampling points over the 24-hour period (Carpenter and Bunney, 1971b). We have recently studied a cyclic manic depressive who exhibited normal periodicity during the depressed phase and an arhythmic series of peaks with no circadian rise during the manic phase. It should be noted that the patient was virtually sleepless for four days during the period of the manic study. Two reported studies on prolonged sleep deprivation (8 1/2-9 days) report normal (Poland, Rubin, Clark and Gouin, 1972) and abnormal periodicity (Slater, Kollar and Pasnau, 1967).

The possible existence of a retino-hypothalamic pathway involved in the regulation of circadian periodicity of corticosteroid levels and the known role of light as a "Zeitgeber" in many rhythmic functions, next leads to a consideration of the role of light and dark (and of wake-sleep) in the initiation of corticosteroid circadian periodicity. Much remains to be done in this field. None of the studies reporting an effect of altered lighting regimens on corticosteroid periodicity has ascertained which parameter of light (its total amount, occurrence at a specific time of day, its wave-length, or some aspect of the light-dark transition) may be the effective stimulus. In animal studies, while there is an association of activity-rest cycles with wake-sleep, there is no evidence that the two are completely synonymous. In any event, to date in studies of corticosteroid periodicity performed under altered lighting regimens, there are no concomittant measurements of activity-wake cycles or of the occurrence of sleep EEG stages to ascertain whether such parameters are altered in association with any alteration seen in corticosteroid periodicity.

A phase shift in corticosteroid periodicity has been reported in animals blinded as adults (Haus, Laktua and Halberg, 1967; Moore and Eichler, 1972) but such studies were carried out only over a 24-hour period. The occurrence of multiple peaks in corticosteroid levels over a 24-hour period in adult animals reared in constant light has been noted by Chiefetz, Gaffud and Dingman (1968) and Scheving and Pauly (1966). We have recently studied (Krieger, 1973a) the effect on corticosteroid periodicity of rearing animals: (a) neonatally under different lighting regimens until adulthood; (b) transfer at different postnatal ages from either normal light-dark alternation to constant light or dark or from neonatal constant light or dark conditions to normal light-dark alternation; or (c) the effect of orbital enucleation at different ages. These studies have indicated that there is no "critical period" in de-

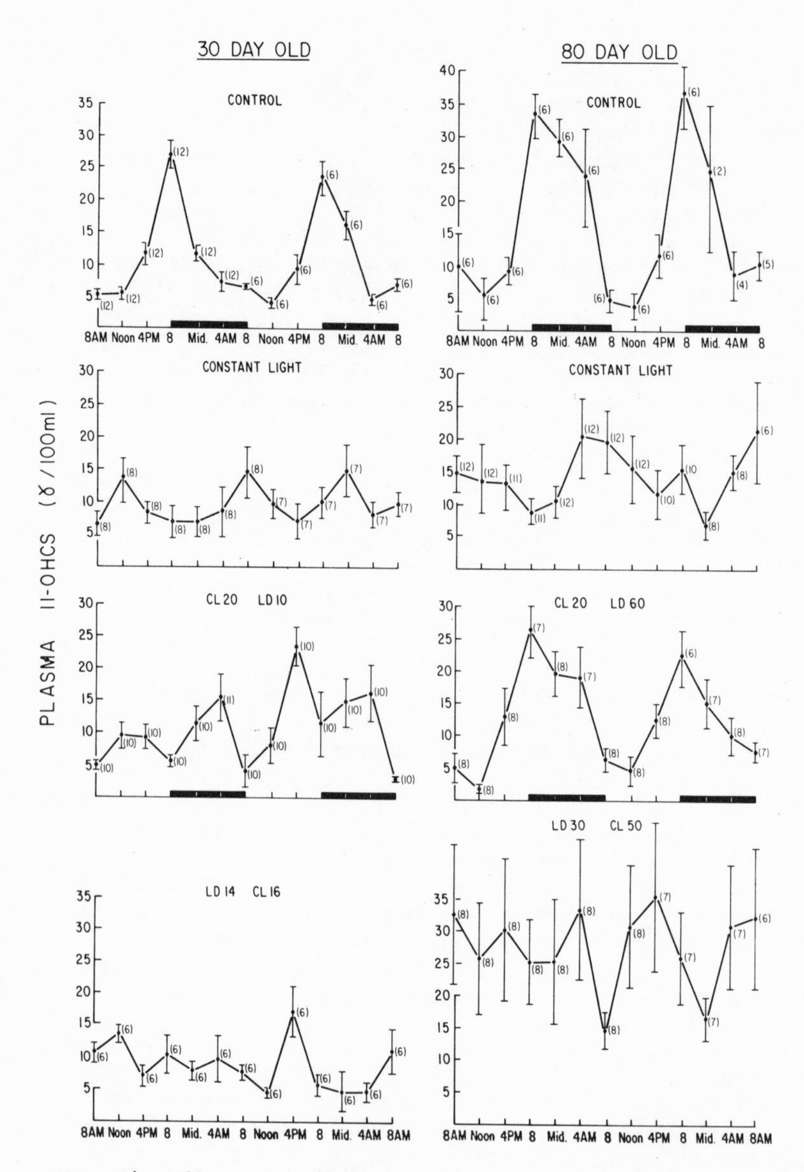

Figure 3A. *Circadian periodicity of plasma 11-hydroxycorticosteroid (11-OHCS) levels in rats raised under varying conditions of constant light. (Group, or "serially independent" sampling at each time point.) Top row of graphs indicates patterns in normal animals raised under 12-hour light, 12-hour dark. Constant light animals reared from birth until indicated age under constant light. CL20 LD10 = reared in constant light till 20 days, normal light-dark until 30 days of*

velopment during which normal light-dark alternation has to be present for such corticosteroid periodicity to subsequently occur nor is there any evidence that such normal periodicity once established can be maintained under abnormal light-dark conditions. Such alteration in periodicity (Figures 3A and 3B) does not appear to be secondary to the development of a free-running state and is not characterized by the flattening of the curve reported in lesioned animals. At present there is only preliminary evidence to relate such alteration in periodicity to concomittant alteration in CNS neurotransmitter levels. From these preliminary observations, it would appear that exposure to constant light at any stage of development is associated with increased mean (average of samples obtained over a 24-hour period) serotonin levels and decreased norepinephrine levels in the amygdalae and decreased serotonin levels and increased norepinephrine levels in the hippocampus.

Studies in the human are at variance with these results. Unlike animals kept in constant light or constant dark, who show abnormal periodicity, normal corticosteroid circadian periodicity has been reported in subjects exposed to either 21 days of constant light (Krieger, Kreuzer and Rizzo, 1969) or 4 (Aschoff, Fatranska, Giedke, Doerr, Stamm and Wisser, 1971) or 10 days (Orth and Island, 1969) of constant darkness. Blind subjects (Krieger and Rizzo, 1971) although showing the normal "early morning rise of plasma corticosteroid levels," manifest abnormal secondary peaks during the course of the day and lack the normal day to day reproducibility of circadian patterns. Similar results have been reported by Orth and Island (1969) and Bodenheimer, Winter and Faiman (1973). The persistence of the early morning rise in corticosteroid levels, despite other abnormalities in the circadian pattern, lends further support to the suggestion that there is a different mechanism responsible for this major circadian rise than for the other corticosteroid elevations noted during the course of 24 hours.

In addition to consideration of a role for light as a "Zeitgeber" conditioning the time of the corticosteroid peak, it is possible that a lights-on signal at any time of the day can initiate a rise in plasma corticosteroid levels. In the constant dark (23 hours) studies cited above (Orth and Island, 1969) an additional corticosteroid rise could be produced by the lights-on period at 6:00-7:00 P.M. Studies by these workers also demonstrated a corticosteroid rise following lights-on at 6:00 P.M. in subjects who underwent light-dark, but not sleep-wake, reversal for 13 days.

From the above, it would appear that the sleep-wake transition might be a more important factor than light-dark in the human with regard to synchronization of corticosteroid circadian periodicity. There is still some question as to whether even this sleep-wake association is only an apparent one and that the corticosteroid rhythm may be a truly

←

age. CL20LD60 = as above, but reared in normal light-dark until 80 days of age. LD14CL16 or LC30CL50 = reared in normal light-dark until 14 or 30 days of age, then in constant light until 30 or 80 days of age respectively.

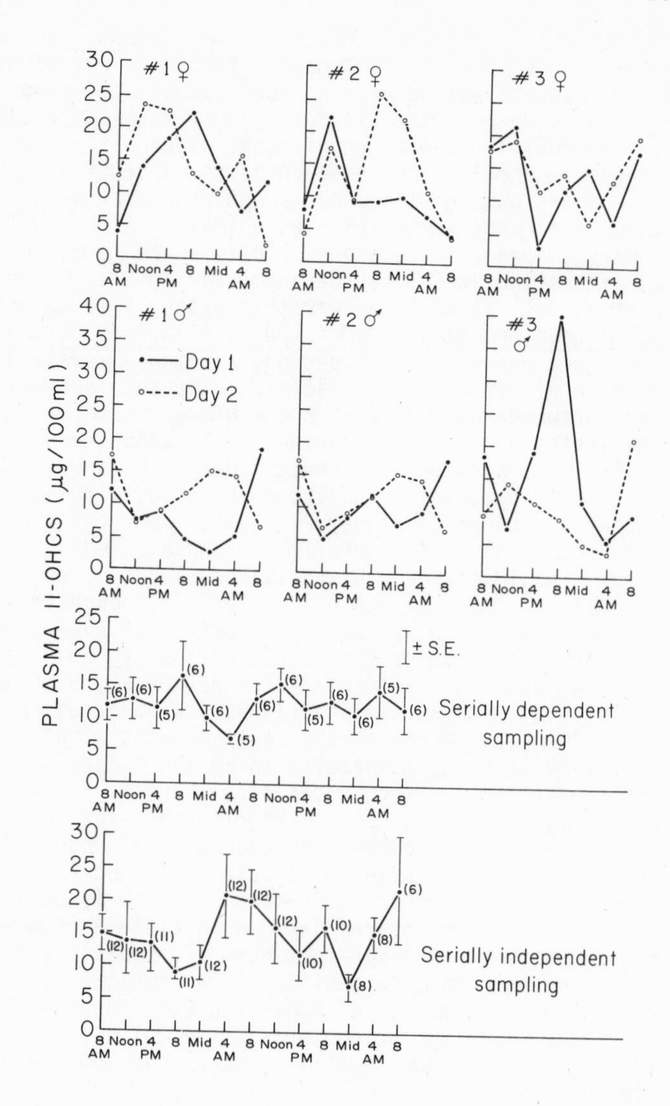

Figure 3B. Circadian periodicity of plasma 11-hydroxycorticosteroid (11-OHCS) levels in six individual 80-day old animals reared from birth in constant light. ("Serially dependent" sampling - all specimens taken sequentially from a given animal.) Dissimilar patterns were obtained in each instance on each of the two study days. The two lower figures contrast the composite pattern derived from averaging these individually obtained serially dependent levels from that derived from group or "serially independent" sampling. (Reproduced by permission, Krieger, 1973a)

endogenous one. Subjects studied after 7 "days" on a 19-hour schedule (one-sixth of each day being spent in sleep), besides showing a rise in corticosteroid levels on awakening (which was the time of lights-on), also showed persistence of the normal early morning circadian rise at a time when there was no dark-light or sleep-wake transition (Orth, Island and Liddle, 1967). These studies also raise the question as to whether corticosteroid periodicity can be "free-running," although as noted above, in some of their studies a basic 24-hour rhythm was present despite evidence of other corticosteroid peaks associated with dark-light or sleep-wake changes. Furthermore, subjects awake for eight consecutive days still show normal corticosteroid periodicit (Poland, Rubin, Clark and Gouin, 1972). On the basis of available evidence it would appear that in the human there is an endogenous 24-hour periodicity of corticosteroid levels, basically related to sleep-wake, in which light can act either as an entraining agent or can independently (outside of the period of major circadian rise) cause elevation of corticosteroid levels.

There have been two other attempts to alter circadian periodicity experimentally that have no human counterparts. One set of experiments involves restriction of water, food, or food and water intake to only a brief period during the normal rest (non-eating-drinking) cycle of an animal (i.e., when corticosteroid levels are at a trough). Johnson and Levine (1973) have noted elevation of plasma corticosteroid levels in this period utilizing such water restriction. We have noted a phase reversal utilizing both food or food and water restriction to this period. Preliminary observations also suggest a phase reversal of serotonin and norepinephrine rhythm in the hippocampus but not in the hypothalamus, of these food and water restricted rats.

Another experimental approach has been to alter the neonatal steroid milieu, in view of reports that development of adult cyclicity of luteinizing hormone release in the female rat depends on the concentration and nature of the gonadal steroid present in the animal <u>immediately</u> after birth (Barraclough, 1961). It was found (Krieger, 1972) that the circadian periodicity of plasma corticosteroid levels was suppressed if corticosteroids were administered systemically between days 2 to 4 of neonatal life but not if they were given between days 12 to 14 of neonatal life (Figure 4). Neonatal administration of testosterone or reserpine had no effect on the subsequent development of corticosteroid periodicity. Other parameters of the CNS-pituitary-adrenal axis (i.e., stress responsiveness, responsiveness to exogenous ACTH) were unaffected by such neonatal steroid treatment. Furthermore, such suppression of periodicity was not a permanent one (unpublished observations), normal periodicity being evident in 80-day old animals who had received corticosteroid between days 2 to 4 of neonatal life.

From the foregoing it appears that circadian adrenal corticosteroid periodicity is a reflection of CNS processes involved in the regulation of periodic CRF and consequently of ACTH release. In some species (including the human) such periodicity appears to be an endogenous one, with the observed time of peaking related to some aspects of the sleep-wake (rest-activity) cycle but also modulated by the light-dark cycle. It is not known whether either of these cycles "drives" the hormonal one or

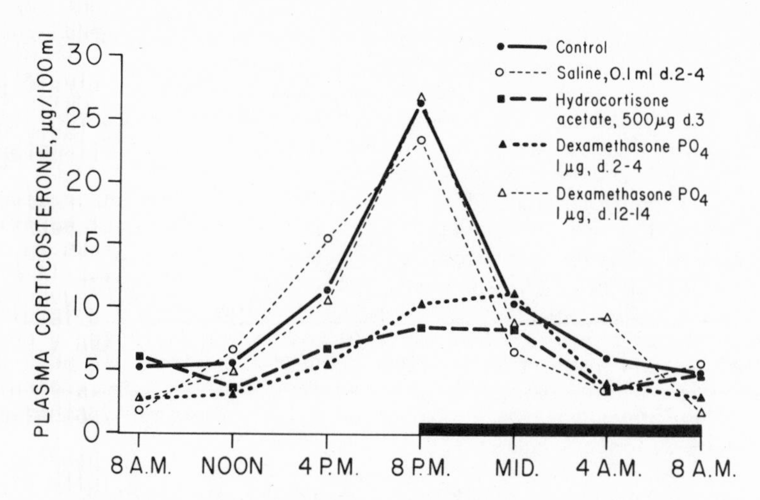

Figure 4. Effect of neonatal administration of corticosteroids on the circadian periodicity of plasma corticosterone concentrations in rats 30 days of age. Black horizontal bar indicates lights off. (Reproduced by permission, Krieger, 1972)

whether all of them are "driven" by a common controller acting independently on each of these variables. In either case, the nature of the "controller" is unknown; one does not know the basis for the observed circadian changes in CNS neurotransmitter content. Likewise, the detailed nature of the anatomical pathways subserving "neural" periodicity is also unknown. Finally, the physiological significance of such periodicity is purely speculative. It is apparent that answers to these and related questions should contribute to fundamental understanding of neural and neuroendocrine processes. The resolution of such questions explains the fascination that investigation of circadian phenomena has had over centuries.

REFERENCES

Ader, R. (1969). Early experiences accelerate maturation of the adrenocortical rhythm. Science 163, 1225-1226.

Allen, C. and Kendall, J. W. (1967). Maturation of the circadian rhythm of plasma corticosterone in the rat. Endocrinology 80, 926-930.

Asano, Y. (1971). The maturation of the circadian rhythm of brain norepinephrine and serotonin in the rat. LIfe Sci. 10, 883-894.

Aschoff, J., Fatranska, M., Giedke, H., Doerr, P., Stamm, D., and Wisser, H. (1971). Human circadian rhythms in continuous darkness: entrainment by social cues. Science 17, 213-215.

Barraclough, C. A. (1961). Production of anovulatory, sterile rats by single injections of testosterone propionate. Endocrinology 68, 62-67.

Besser, G. M., Cullen, D. R., Irvine, W. J., Ratcliff, J. G. , and Landon, J. (1971). Immunoreactive corticotrophin levels in adrenocortical insufficiency. Brit. Med. J. 1, 374-376.

Besser, G. M., Orth, D. N., Nicholson, W. E., Byyny, R. L., Abe, K., and Woodham, J. P. (1971). Dissociation of the disappearance of bioactive and radioimmunoreactive ACTH from plasma in man. J. Clin. Endocrinol. Metab. 32, 595-608.

Bodenheimer, S., Winter, J. S. D. and Faiman, C. (1973). Diurnal rhythms of serum gonadotropins, testosterone, estradiol and cortisol in blind men. J. Clin. Endocrinol. Metab. 37, 472-475.

Bridges, P. K. and Jones, M. T. (1966). The diurnal rhythm of plasma cortisol concentration in depression. Brit. J. Psychiat. 112, 1257-1261.

Carpenter, W. T., Jr. and Bunney, W. E., Jr. (1971a). Adrenal cortical activity in depressive illness. Amer. J. Psychiat. 128, 31-40.

Carpenter, W. T., Jr. and Bunney, W. E., Jr. (1971b). Diurnal rhythm of cortisol in mania. Arch. Gen. Psychiat. 25, 270-273.

Cheifetz, P., Gaffud, N., and Dingman, J. F. (1968). Effects of bilateral adrenalectomy and continuous light on the circadian rhythm of corticotropin in female rats. Endocrinology 82, 1117-1124.

DeLacerda, L., Kowarski, A., and Migeon, C. J. (1973). Diurnal variation of the metabolic clearance rate of cortisol. Effect on measurement of cortisol production rate. J. Clin. Endocrinol. Metab. 36, 1043-1049.

DeMoor, P., Heirwegh, K., Hermans, J. K., and Declerck-Raskin, M. (1962). Protein binding of corticoids studied by gel filtration. J. Clin. Invest. 41, 816.

Doe, R. P., Vennes, J. A., and Flink, E. B. (1960). Diurnal variation of 17-hydroxycorticosteroids, sodium, potassium, magnesium and creatinine in normal subjects and in cases of adrenal insufficiency and Cushing's syndrome. J. Clin. Endocrinol. Metab. 20, 253-265.

Dusseau, W. and Meier, A. H. (1971). Diurnal and seasonal variations of plasma adrenal steroid hormone in the white-throated sparrow, *Zonotrichia albicollis*. Gen. Comp. Endocrinol. 16, 399-408.

Franks, R. (1967). Diurnal variation of plasma 17-OHCS in children. J. Clin. Endocrinol. Metab. 27, 75-78.

Fullerton, D. T., Wenzel, F. J., Lohrenz, F. N. and Fahs, H. (1968). Circadian rhythm of adrenal cortical activity in depression. Arch. Gen. Psychiat. 19, 674-682.

Graber, A. L., Givens, J., Nicholson, W., Island, D. P., and Liddle, D. W. (1965). Persistence of diurnal rhythmicity in plasma ACTH concentrations in cortisol deficient patients. J. Clin. Endocrinol. Metab. 25, 804-807.

Greer, M. A., Panton, P., and Allen, C. F. (1972). Relationship of nychthermeral cycles of running activity and plasma corticosterone concentration following basal hypothalamic isolation. Horm. Behav. 3, 289-295.

Guillemin, R., Dear, W. E., and Liebilt, R. A. (1959). Nychthemeral variations in plasma free corticosteroid levels of the rat. Proc. Soc. Exp. Biol. Med. 101, 394-395.
Halász, B., Slusher, M. A., and Gorski, R. A. (1967). Adrenocorticotrophic hormone secretion in rats after partial or total deafferentiation of the medical basal hypothalamus. Neuroendocrinology 2, 43-55.
Halberg, F. (1969). Chronobiology. Annu. Rev. Physiol. 31, 675-725.
Hanin, I., Massarelli, R., and Costa, E. (1970). Acetylcholine concentrations in rat brain: diurnal oscillation. Science 170, 341-342.
Haus, E., Lakatua, D., and Halberg, F. (1967). The internal timing of several circadian rhythms in the blinded mouse. Exp. Med. Surg. 25, 7-45.
Hellman, L., Nakada, F., Curti, J., Weitzman, E. D., Kream, J., Roffward, H., Ellman, S., Fukushima, D. K., and Gallagher, T. F. (1970). Cortisol is secreted episodically by normal man. J. Clin. Endocrinol. Metab. 30, 411-422.
Hiroshige, T. and Sakakura, M. (1971). Circadian rhythm of corticotropin releasing activity in the hypothalamus of normal and adrenalectomized rats. Neuroendocrinology 7, 25-36.
Hiroshige, T. and Sato, T. (1970). Postnatal development of circadian rhythm of corticotropin-releasing activity in the rat hypothalamus. Endocrinol. Jap. 17, 1-6.
Jailer, J. W. (1950). The maturation of the pituitary-adrenal axis in the newborn rat. Endocrinology 46, 420-425.
Johnson, J. T. and Levine, S. (1973). Influence of water deprivation on adrenocortical rhythms. Neuroendocrinology 11, 268-273.
Krieger, D. T. (1973a). Effect of ocular enucleation and altered lighting regimens at various ages on the circadian periodicity of plasma corticosteroid levels in the rat. Endocrinology 93, 1077-1091.
Krieger, D. T. (1973b). Pathophysiology of central nervous system regulation of anterior pituitary function. In: *Biology of Brain Dysfunction*, Volume II, in press, Plenum Press, New York.
Krieger, D. T. (1973c). Neurotransmitter regulation of ACTH release. Mt. Sinai J. Med. New York 40, 302-304.
Krieger, D. T. (1972). Circadian corticosteroid periodicity: critical period for abolition by neonatal injection of corticosteroid. Science 178, 1205-1207.
Krieger, D. T. (1969). Factors influencing the circadian periodicity of adrenal steroid levels. Trans. N.Y. Acad. Sci. 32, 316-329.
Krieger, D. T. (1961). Diurnal pattern of plasma 17-hydroxycorticosteroids in pretectal and temporal lobe disease. J. Clin. Endocrinol. Metab. 21, 695-698.
Krieger, D. T. and Glick, S. M. (1972). Growth hormone and cortisol responsiveness in Cushing's syndrome: relation to a possible central nervous system etiology. Amer. J. Med. 52, 25-40.
Krieger, D. T. and Rizzo, F. (1971). Circadian periodicity of plasma 11-hydroxycorticosteroid levels in subjects with partial and absent light perception. Neuroendocrinology 8, 165-179.

Krieger, D. T., Allen, W., Rizzo, F., and Krieger, H. P. (1971). Characterization of the normal pattern of plasma corticosteroid levels. J. Clin. Endocrinol. Metab. 32, 266-284.

Krieger, D. T. and Rizzo, F. (1969). Circadian periodicity of plasma 17-OHCS: mediation by serotonin dependent pathways. Amer. J. Physiol. 217, 1703-1707.

Krieger, D. T., Kreuzer, J., and Rizzo, F. A. (1969). Constant light: effect on circadian pattern and phase reversal of steroid and electrolyte levels in man. J. Clin. Endocrinol. Metab. 29, 1634-1638.

Krieger, D. T., Silverberg, A. I., Rizzo, F., and Krieger, H. P. (1968). Abolition of circadian periodicity of plasma 17-OHCS levels in the cat. Am. J. Physiol. 215, 959-967.

Krieger, D. T. and Krieger, H. P. (1967). The effect of short-term administration of CNS-acting drugs on the circadian variation of the plasma 17-OHCS in normal subjects. Neuroendocrinology 2, 232-246.

Krieger, D. T. and Krieger, H. P. (1966). Circadian variation of the plasma 17-hydroxycorticosteroids in central nervous system disease. J. Clin. Endocrinol. Metab. 26, 929-940.

Lengvari, I. and Halász, B. (1973). Evidence for a diurnal fluctuation in plasma corticosterone levels after fornix transection in the rat. Neuroendocrinology 11, 191-196.

Marti, H., Studer, H., Dettweiler, W., and Rohner, R. (1969). Persistence of a physiological circadian rhythm of plasma-free 11-hydroxycorticosteroid in totally fasting obese subjects. Experientia 25, 320-321.

Matsuyama, H., Ruhmann-Wennhold, A., Johnson, L. R., and Nelson, D. H. (1972). Disappearance rates of exogenous and endogenous ACTH from rat plasma measured by bioassay and radioimmunoassay. Metab. Clin. Exp. 21, 30-35.

Migeon, C. J., Tyler, F. H., Mahoney, J. P., Florentin, A. A., Castle, H., Bliss, E. L., and Samuels, L. T. (1956). The diurnal variation of plasma levels and urinary excretion of 17-hydroxycorticosteroids in normal subjects, night workers and blind subjects in man. J. Clin. Endocrinol. Metab. 16, 622-633.

Milkovíc, K. and Milkovíc, S. (1966). Adrenocorticotropic hormone secretion in the fetus and infant. In: *Neuroendocrinology* (Martini, L. and Ganong, W. F., eds.), Volume I, pp. 371-405, Academic Press, New York.

Moberg, G. P., Scapagnini, V., deGroot, J., and Ganong, W. F. (1971). Effect of sectioning the fornix on diurnal fluctuation in plasma corticosterone levels in the rat. Neuroendocrinology 7, 11-15.

Moore, R. Y. and Eichler, V. B. (1972). Loss of a circadian adrenal corticosterone rhythm following suprachiasmatic lesions in the rat. Brain Res. 42, 201-206.

Moore, R. Y. and Lenn, N. J. (1972). A retinohypothalamic projection in the rat. J. Comp. Neurol. 146, 1-14

Nugent, C. A., Eik-Nes, K., Kent, H. S., Samuels, L. T., and Tyler, F. H. (1960). A possible explanation for Cushing's syndrome associated with adrenal hyperplasia. J. Clin. Endocrinol. Metab. 20, 1259-1268.

Orth, D. N. and Island, D. P. (1969). Light synchronization of the circadian rhythm in plasma cortisol (17-OHCS) concentration in man. J. Clin. Endocrinol. Metab. 29, 479-486.
Orth, D. N., Island, D. P., and Liddle, G. W. (1967). Experimental alteration of the circadian rhythm in plasma cortisol (17-OHCS) concentration in man. J. Clin. Endocrinol. Metab. 27, 549-555.
Palka, A., Coyer, D., and Critchlow, V. (1969). Effects of isolation of medial basal hypothalamus on pituitary-adrenal and pituitary-ovarian functions. Neuroendocrinology 5, 333-349.
Perkoff, G. T., Eik-Nes, K., Nugent, C. A., Fred, H. L., Nimer, R. A., Rush, L., Samuels, L. T., and Tyler, F. H. (1959). Studies of the diurnal variation of plasma 17-hydroxycorticosteroids. J. Clin. Endocrinol. Metab. 16, 432-443.
Poland, R. E., Rubin, R. T., Clark, B. R., and Gouin, P. R. (1972). Circadian patterns of urine 17-OHC and VMA secretion during sleep deprivation. Dis. Nerv. Syst. 33, 456-458.
Reis, D. J., Corvelli, A., and Conners, J. (1969). Circadian and ultradian rhythms of serotonin regionally in cat brain. J. Pharmacol. Exp. Ther. 167, 328-333.
Reis, D. J., Weinbren, M., and Corvelli, A. (1968). A circadian rhythm of norepinephrine regionally in cat brain: its relationship to environmental lighting and to regional diurnal variations in brain serotonin. J. Pharmacol. Exp. Ther. 164, 135-145.
Sachar, E. J., Hellman, L., Roffwarg, H. P., Halpern, F. S., Fukushima, D. K., and Gallagher, T. F. (1973). Disrupted 24-hour patterns of cortisol secretion in psychotic depression. Arch. Gen. Psychiat. 28, 19-24.
Scheving, L. E. and Pauly, J. E. (1966). Effect of light on corticosterone levels in plasma of rats. Am. J. Physiol. 210, 1112-1117.
Sholiton, L. J., Werk, E. E., Jr., and Marnell, R. T. (1961). Diurnal variation of adrenocortical function in non-endocrine disease states. Metab. Clin. Exp. 10, 632-646.
Singley, J. A. and Chavin, W. (1971). Cortisol levels of normal goldfish and response to osmotic change. Am. Zool. 11, 653 (Abstract).
Slater, G. G., Kollar, E. J., and Pasnau, R. O. (1967). Plasma corticoids cholesterol and glucose changes in men during 204 hours of sleep deprivation. Fed. Proc. 26, 484.
Slusher, M. A. (1964). Effect of chronic hypothalamic lesions on diurnal and stress corticosteroid levels. Amer. J. Physiol. 206, 1161-1164.
Stephan, F. K. and Zucker, I. (1972). Circadian rhythms in drinking behavior and locomotor activity of rats are eliminated by hypothalamic lesions. Proc. Nat. Acad. Sci., U.S.A. 69, 1583-1586.
Takebe, K., Sakakura, M., and Mashimo, K. (1972). Continuance of diurnal rhythmicity of CRF activity in hypophysectomized rats. Endocrinology 90, 1515-1520.
Tucci, J. R., Albacete, R. A., and Martin, M. M. (1966). Effect of liver disease upon steroid circadian rhythms in man. Gastroenterology 50, 637-644.
Ungar, F. (1964). In vitro studies of adrenal-pituitary circadian rhythms in the mouse. Ann. N.Y. Acad. Sci. 117, 374-385.
Vernikos-Danellis, J., Leach, C. S., Winget, C. M., Rambaut, P. C., and Mack, P. B. (1972). Thyroid and adrenal cortical rhythmicity during bed rest. J. Appl. Physiol. 33, 644-648.

DISCUSSION AFTER DR. KRIEGER'S PAPER

Dr. Craig

In one of your earlier slides you showed some sleep and wake patterns (see Figures 1 and 2). Have you seen any work where they have used exercise at any point of the day in patients and what effects this would have? It has been shown that if you use strenuous exercise, you will first increase (3 weeks) corticoid levels and then decrease (6 weeks) corticoid levels (Korenskaya, 1967; Suzuki et al., 1967).

Dr. Krieger

The only study I know is the study that Vernikos-Danellis et al. (1971) did on patients who were kept in bed for periods of 90 days and they found that whether patients did isometric exercise in bed or whether the patients were completely prone with no exercise there was no alteration of the normal circadian pattern.

Dr. Craig

I've seen those studies and I think the reason they didn't see any effects is because they did not use strenuous exercise, but non-strenuous, as they define it, which doesn't seem to have as much of an effect.

Dr. Krieger

I know of no studies of periodicity, for example, in athletes after a period of stressful exercise who were sampled subsequently during the night.

Dr. Reiter

Dr. Krieger, what is the time sequence for the disappearance of the corticosterone rhythm in the constant light-exposed animals as opposed to the blinded animals?

Dr. Krieger

Obviously, there are all kinds of gradations that one can do. The shortest interval studied was 16 days after introduction of the stimulus. In other words, in adult animals who had normal periodicity, and were put into constant light or constant dark, periodicity was disrupted (in group studies) when measured 16 days later.

Dr. Reiter

You mentioned that in neither case did you have ideas concerning mechanisms involved. I think it's quite possible that in blinded experimental animals and in the blind human as well, the altered corticosterone rhythm may be related to a stimulated pineal gland. A paper was presented last year at the International Endocrine Meetings in Washington by Jacobs and Kendall (1972) which supports this conclusion. They reported that in chronically blinded rats the afternoon rise in plasma corticosterone was depressed and that it was partially restored by pinealectomy. I suspect the rhythm persisted in the pinealectomized animals but became free-running, so they didn't see the normal afternoon rise.

Dr. Krieger

Now this is something in which we're interested, but I have no additional information. One part of our protocol was to add pinealectomy, but the number of permutations is such that we haven't done this yet.

Dr. Reiter

The only thing that speaks against the theory stated above is the paper by Hiroshige et al. (1973) which you mentioned. They examined the circadian variation in CRF content of the hypothalamus. They also included animals that were superior cervical ganglionectomized. Of course, this procedure functionally denervates the pineal gland. They found it to have no effect on the circadian variation of CRF within the hypothalamus. However, they kept their animals under alternating light-dark conditions.

Dr. Krieger

And it may very well be that you need the stimulus to show the effect.

Dr. Kitay

Dorothy, I was trying to recall some data that I remember reading this past year about steady-state secretion rate of cortisol in man throughout a 24-hour period.

Dr. Krieger

You're talking about Hellman's group?

Dr. Kitay

Yes. If I remember correctly, they did not show the same kind of variation.

Dr. Krieger

No, they showed periods in which there was zero secretion and periods in which there was markedly increased secretion.

Dr. Kitay

Was it cyclic?

Dr. Krieger

They attempted to say that this occurred with a periodicity of approximately 90 minutes. Their data really don't seem to support such an exact cycle length and neither does ours.

Dr. Kitay

I am trying to relate the variations in plasma cortisol in your human subjects to biological half-time and then speculating back to what the steady-state secretion rate might be during the day. I wonder if one were to utilize steady-state secretion rate as the criterion rather than plasma cortisol, then one might come up with entirely different answers. We have tried to measure steady-state corticosterone secretion rates at two different times in the day. While plasma corticosterone does indeed vary, steady-state secretion rate may not. There are several reasons that one could ascribe to this lack of variation. One is a hormonally regulated volume of distribution; another is a hormonally regulated set-point difference.

Dr. Krieger

How were you measuring steady-state secretion rate?

Dr. Kitay

Injection of labelled steroid, measurements over an appropriate period, extrapolating back to zero time, and the appropriate calculations.

Dr. Krieger

Hellman et al. (1970) in their experiments albeit, on one subject, did essentially the same sort of studies and all I can say is that they had differences in steady-state secretion based on that. With regard to half-life determinations, varying half-lives for cortisol were obtained based on whether or not one inferred continued secretion following a burst of secretion. In other words, from their experiments with labelled cortisol they inferred that with certain spurts of secretion there was absolute cut-off of secretion after that spurt. With other spurts there was also some fall-off, but the apparent half-life was prolonged because there was continued low level secretion of cortisol.

Dr. Kitay

The point I want to make is that if one is attempting to look at a coupled mechanism that starts in the brain and is transmitted via CRF and ACTH to steroid secretion, then shouldn't one really have to show this as an effect of ACTH on the adrenal in the form of smooth changes or cyclic changes in steroid secretion rates.

Dr. Krieger

One should and this becomes a very difficult problem. If we do sampling, say every five minutes, we get a plasma adrenal corticosteroid pattern and a plasma ACTH pattern that are pretty much in parallel. Then we may suddenly get spurts of ACTH secretion where we find nothing happening with plasma cortisol levels. Now, I'm not sure what this represents, and this is something we are puzzling about. There are two possible suggestions and there may be many, many more. One is that the rate of presentation of ACTH to the adrenal varies. In other words, there may be some variation in adrenal blood flow during all these sequential samplings so that what we're measuring as changes in plasma ACTH levels are not seen in the same way by the adrenal. The other suggestion may be even more problematical. Is the ACTH we're measuring by immunoassay biologically active ACTH? What we're embarking on right now is to try to simultaneously determine the immunoassayable and the bioassayable levels of ACTH as well as plasma cortisol levels before we can make any correlation between plasma ACTH and plasma cortisol levels. There is some suggestive evidence that under different stimuli the kind of ACTH released is not the same.

Dr. Dellmann

You showed in your first slide (Figure 1) the rise in plasma corticosteroids between four and six o'clock in the morning, I think, when the subjects got up at eight o'clock in the morning. Now I assume they had a very periodic sleep, that is, they got up every morning at eight o'clock. What happens if you disturb this sleep pattern? When does the rise in plasma corticosteroids occur?

Dr. Krieger

This varies. The rise in steroids is not as locked into when you go to sleep and exactly when you wake up as, say the rise in growth hormone. So that I think we have to talk about, for example, two different kinds of sleep-associated hormonal release. Plasma growth hormone levels rise an hour and a half after you go to sleep. Now, if you go to sleep at ten o'clock you'll get the rise, say at 11:30 to 12:00; if you go to bed at 12:00 midnight you'll get the rise at 1:30 or 2:00 A.M.; and if you then wake the person up and you let them go to sleep again you'll get another rise in growth hormone 1-1/2 hours later. The "sleep-associated" plasma cortisol pattern is different. In other words, you can go to sleep at 10:00 P.M. or you can go to sleep at 1:00 A.M., and you'll still get the same early morning rise in plasma cortisol levels in both instances. However, if you delay the time of getting out of bed, keeping the subject in the dark, to some extent you delay the time of the corticosteroid peak, even though the actual rise still starts pretty much at the same time in the early morning as previously. Now, if someone doesn't go to sleep (this hasn't been done in too many instances, one reported instance had to do with some studies Dr. Halberg did on himself and some other subjects where they were up two nights around the clock with no sleep), there still is a normal periodicity There is one abstract that I'm aware of, reporting on subjects who were kept awake for eight consecutive days where both they and their corticosteroid patterns went totally beserk. I think when you have complete sleep deprivation you're running into other factors other than the lack of sleep. So, I'm glad you brought the point up because even though there is a sleep-associated rhythm it doesn't seem to be associated with a specific stage of sleep and with a particular hour to hour correlation as to either when you go to sleep or when you wake up. Now, if you were to arise regularly, say very early in the morning, i.e., at 4:00 A.M., then your steroid peak would occur earlier than 4:00 A.M. and cortisol levels might begin to rise at one or two in the morning.

Dr. Dellmann
Which of the neurotransmitters is correlated in its periodicity with CRF release?

Dr. Krieger
I wish I knew.

DISCUSSION REFERENCES

Hellman, L., Nakada, F., Curti, J., Weitzman, E. D., Kream, J., Roffward, H., Ellman, S., Fukushima, D. K., and Gallagher, T. F. (1970). J. Clin. Endocrinol. 30, 411-422.
Hiroshige, T., Abe, K., Wada, S., and Kanek, M. (1973). Neuroendocrinology 11, 306-320.
Jacobs, J. J., and Kendall, J. W. (1972). In: *IV International Congress of Endocrinology, Abstracts of Short Communications*, p. 53, Excerpta Medica, Amsterdam.
Korenskaya, E. F. (1967). Probl. Endokrinol. (Mosk) 13, 65-68.
Suzuki, T., Otsuka, K., Matsui, H., Ohakuzi, S., Sakai, K., and Harada, Y. (1967). Endocrinology 80, 1148-1151.
Vernikos-Danellis, J., Leach, C. S., Winget, C. M., Rambaut, P. C., and Mack, P. B. (1971). J. Appl. Physiol. 33, 644-648.

SUBJECT INDEX